Conservative Treatment of Male Urinary Incontinence and Erectile Dysfunction

Conservative Treatment of Male Urinary Incontinence and Erectile Dysfunction

A textbook for physiotherapists, nurses and doctors

GRACE DOREY MSc MCSP

Specialist Continence Physiotherapist, Somerset Nuffield Hospital, Taunton and North Devon District NHS Trust, Barnstaple

W
WHURR PUBLISHERS
LONDON AND PHILADELPHIA

© 2001 Whurr Publishers
First published 2001 by
Whurr Publishers Ltd
19b Compton Terrace, London N1 2UN, England and
325 Chestnut Street, Philadelphia PA 19106, USA

Reprinted 2002

British Library Cataloguing in Publication Data
A catalogue record for this book is available from the
British Library.

ISBN: 1 86156 302 7

Printed and bound in the UK by Athenaeum Press Ltd,
Gateshead, Tyne & Wear

Contents

Preface

This book is written primarily for those specialist continence physiotherapists who treat female continence problems but who are unsure of the treatment for male patients with lower urinary tract symptoms. It will be a useful reference tool for urology nurses, continence specialist nurses and continence advisors; and those medical students, student nurses and physiotherapy students suddenly finding themselves on a urology placement. It will provide a greater knowledge of conservative treatment in this speciality for urologists and GPs. Where possible, the information is based on the current literature, even though this is sparse in some areas. The avid reader and the questioning research student may find the references provide further, fascinating and more in-depth reading.

Background details concerning the prevalence of male lower urinary tract symptoms, the anatomy and physiology of the pelvic floor and the physiology of the continence mechanism are provided in order to explain the dysfunction that can occur.

The different prostatic conditions are covered in detail, plus the range of standardised medical and surgical investigations and treatments. The various types of incontinence are explained, and a comprehensive classification of male urinary incontinence tabulated. The subjective and objective physiotherapy assessment is covered chronologically to enable the clinician to conduct a meaningful investigation and arrive at a logical diagnosis.

Recommended conservative treatment options are provided for each type of incontinence, with a range of patient advice added for completeness. Treatment outcomes, which may vary considerably, are discussed.

Following the treatment chapter, there are case studies, which provide question and answer sessions for the student to check their knowledge base, and for the more experienced, to act as an aide memoire. There are two chapters on the aetiology and conservative treatment of erectile dysfunction which are based on an extensive literature search. The appendix includes subjective and objective continence assessment forms and examples of patient information sheets, and a list of definitions and abbreviations to explain the medical jargon is provided, to help those readers who do not have a medical background or are unfamiliar with some of the more obscure urology terminology.

This is the book that I would have welcomed before embarking on my MSc. It contains information that I have spent three years gathering, analysing and compiling, and I hope you will find it interesting, informative and a useful reference source. Good luck with your studies.

Grace Dorey MSc MCSP
June 2001

Acknowledgements

I sincerely thank the clinical reviewers for their contribution, wisdom and considerable support. I would also like to thank my daughter Claire for her accurate anatomical illustrations.

Clinical reviewers

Mrs Jane Dixon MCSP
Professor Roger Feneley FRCS
Mrs Jeanette Haslam MPhil MCSP
Dr Katherine Moore PhD RN

Illustrator

Claire Dorey BA (Hons)

Dedication

To my physiotherapy colleague Claire, who sent me my first male urology patient, and who caused me to explore this subject in greater depth. To my first male urology patient, a delightful man who must remain anonymous, but who patiently waited for me to research the subject.

CHAPTER 1

Lower urinary tract symptoms

Key points

- Male lower urinary tract symptoms include nocturia, frequency, urgency, urge incontinence, stress incontinence and post-micturition dribble.
- Moderate to severe lower urinary tract symptoms occur in 29–51% of men in the UK aged 50 years and over.
- The International Prostate Symptom Score gives identical readings for men with and without obstruction and for age-matched women.

Male lower urinary tract symptoms

Male lower urinary tract symptoms (LUTS) include nocturia, frequency, urgency, urge incontinence, stress incontinence, post-micturition dribble, heistancy, weak stream, intermittency, pain, dysuria and haematuria (Neal, 1990; Chute *et al*, 1993; Hunter *et al*, 1996; de la Rosette *et al*, 1998; Kortmann *et al*, 1999; Dorey, 2000f) (see Table 1.1). In elderly men many of the symptoms are caused by benign prostatic hyperplasia (BPH), but up to one-third of symptoms have other causes such as detrusor instability and detrusor underactivity (Kortmann *et al*, 1999). Lower urinary tract problems contribute to social and psychological problems which may severely affect quality of life.

Former 'prostatic' symptoms

Abrams (1994) divided LUTS in men into voiding and filling symptoms, as shown in Table 1.2.

1

Table 1.1 Lower urinary tract symptoms in men

Nocturia
Frequency
Urgency
Urge incontinence
Nocturnal enuresis
Stress incontinence
Post-micturition dribble
Incomplete emptying
Acute retention
Weak stream
Hesitancy/straining
Intermittency
Terminal dribble
Dysuria
Bladder pain
Burning
Haematuria

Table 1.2 Bladder filling and voiding symptoms in men (Abrams, 1994 reproduced with permission)

Filling symptoms	Voiding symptoms
Frequency	Hesitancy
Urgency	Poor stream
Urge incontinence	Straining
Nocturia	Incomplete emptying
	Intermittency
	Terminal dribble

Lower urinary tract symptoms used to be synonymous with 'prostatic' symptoms. In 1994, Abrams reported that older men with LUTS were described as having symptoms of BPH. The following year, he stated that the term 'prostatism' should be abandoned, and the term 'lower urinary tract symptoms' should be used instead (Abrams, 1995). More weight was given to the thinking that LUTS were not just symptoms of prostatism when Abrams (1995) stated that the International–Prostate Symptom Score (I-PSS) gave identical readings in men with and without obstruction and also in age-matched women (Lepor and Grace, 1993). LUTS were not necessarily related to urodynamically proven bladder outlet obstruction (BOO) or histologically proven BPH (Abrams, 1994). Indeed, Scafer *et al* (1988) stated that one-third of men did not have outflow obstruction but had detrusor underactivity as the cause of their reduced stream. Symptoms could be present before or after BOO and also before and after surgery to remove the obstruction (Neal, 1990). Neal found that 25% of men complained of frequency, urgency and occasionally incontinence after transurethral resection of prostate (TURP) and that most had suffered symptoms before surgery. Symptoms such as nocturia and straining were found to exist similarly in elderly women (Jolleys et al, 1993).

Research implicated that BOO could exacerbate LUTS or cause a variety of bladder changes which may result in new LUTS. Obstruction from prostate cancer may also cause obstructive (voiding) and irritative (filling) symptoms in the later stages although this cancer is usually symptom free in the early stages. There is no clear relationship between prostate size and symptoms (Simpson et al, 1996). When the urethral obstruction is removed by either TURP or radical prostatectomy, incontinence may ensue. The cause may be sphincteric incompetence (Foote et al, 1991) or filling symptoms or a combination of both. Interestingly, the LUTS listed in Table 1.2 include urge incontinence as being a problem of filling, but other symptoms such as stress incontinence or post-micturition dribble are not listed by Abrams (1994).

Prostate symptom scores

Urologists and general practitioners use prostate symptom scores in order to assess the severity of prostatic symptoms. This will determine the need for surgery for the obstruction. Various unvalidated prostate symptom scores have been used previously but these were replaced in 1991 by the International–Prostate Symptom Score (I-PSS) validated by the International Continence Society (ICS).

Unvalidated questionnaires

There have been three unvalidated questionnaires from the USA. Both the Boyarsky Score (Boyarsky et al, 1977) and the Madsen–Iversen Score (Madsen and Iversen, 1983) were designed to be completed by doctors and were never validated. The Maine Medical Assessment Program (MMAP) Instrument (Fowler et al, 1988), although not validated, was the first questionnaire to be designed for completion by patients.

Validated questionnaires

The Danish Prostatic Symptom Score (DAN-PSS-1) (Hald et al, 1991; Hansen et al, 1995) contains a symptom/symptom-botherness section and a sexual questionnaire. There are 24 questions, which are considered to be confusing to elderly patients.

The Bolognese Symptom Questionnaire for BPH (Bolognese *et al*, 1992) contains a symptom section, a symptom-bothersomeness section and one question on urination. It was constructed for a clinical trial assessing the effect of finasteride, but otherwise has not been used.

The I-PSS (Cockett *et al*, 1991; Barry *et al*, 1992) was derived from the American Urologic Association (AUA) symptom score with the addition of a condition-specific quality-of-life question. The I-PSS is the most frequently used of the questionnaires. In order to assess the severity of LUTS patients report if they have suffered from the following symptoms within the last month:

incomplete emptying
frequency
intermittency
urgency
weak stream
straining
nocturia

Each question is scored 0–5, giving a possible total of 35:

0   not at all
1   less than 1 time in 5
2   less than half the time
4   more than half the time
5   almost always

Patients are also asked to rate their quality of life due their to urinary symptoms from the following seven categories:

1   delighted
2   pleased
3   mostly satisfied
4   mixed about equally satisfied and dissatisfied
5   mostly dissatisfied
6   unhappy
7   terrible

Surgery may be appropriate for men with a score of 20 or over. This was confirmed by Cliff *et al* (1997) following a trial of 3442 men aged over 40 years.

When Abrams (1995) found that the I-PSS gave identical readings for men with and without obstruction and for age-matched women, he advocated 'watchful waiting' as an alternative to surgery. Also, a 2 year group study in Canada reported that placebo therapy rapidly produced a significant improvement in Q_{max} (maximum urinary flow rate) and symptoms of BPH (Nickel, 1998). Patients may have previously undergone TURP because urinary symptoms such as frequency, urgency, nocturia, and therefore poor quality of life, gave a high I-PSS score. The former 'prostatic' symptoms of frequency, urgency and nocturia could still be present after surgery.

Because some of the urinary symptoms were considered to be unrelated to prostatic outflow obstruction, Donovan *et al* (1996) compiled the ICS*male* Questionnaire which was considered to be a more accurate way to assess male urinary symptoms. Unfortunately, it does not contain questions related to symptoms such as incontinence which may develop following treatment. The ICS*male* Questionnaire contains questions on 20 urinary symptoms, 19 of which have an additional question to ascertain the degree of bother that they cause. It is easy for the patient to complete. The questions on frequency and nocturia demonstrate reasonable agreement with frequency/volume (F/V) charts, but there is a poor relationship between questions assessing stream and the results of uroflowmetry. This questionnaire was shown to have good internal consistency and good test–retest reliability. It was considered a breakthrough for assessing the severity of LUTS.

There is still controversy as to the need for a prostate symptom score. In a prospective study of 126 consecutive men with LUTS, Vestey and Hinchcliffe (1998) compared the I-PSS to a 7 day F/V chart. They found that 64% of men overestimated their frequency and 47% their nocturia on the I-PSS questionnaires. Half the scores revealed nocturnal polyuria (>33% urinary output during bedtime hours), with 11% of men producing more than 50% of their output at night. There was no correlation between the I-PSS and post-void residual volumes for incomplete bladder emptying, and no correlation between the I-PSS and maximum flow rates for patients with a weak stream. They concluded that the F/V chart, in combination with flowmetry and post-void residuals, answered the I-PSS questions more objectively and in more detail than the I-PSS

questionnaire. In addition, the F/V chart provided important information on nocturnal output, co-morbidity and social habits. They recommended the routine use of F/V charts for the assessment of male LUTS.

Quality of life

Quality of life has been linked to the World Health Organisation definition of health (WHO, 1978), which was defined as a state of physical,
emotional and social well-being, and not just the absence of disease or
infirmity. The quality of life is subjective. Some condition specific questionnaires assess the quality of life and some the bothersomeness of symptoms for men with LUTS (see Table 1.3).

Table 1.3 Condition-specific questionnaires and quality of life questionnaires (Donovan,
1999 reproduced with permission)

Questionnaire	Reference
Condition-specific:	
AUA bother index	Barry *et al* (1992)
DAN-PSS-1	Hald *et al* (1991)
ICS*male*	Donovan *et al* (1996)
Quality of life:	
BPH Impact Index	Barry *et al* (1995)
Veterans Affairs	Anonymous (1993)
Olmstead County Index	Girman *et al* (1994)
BPH QL	Epstein *et al* (1992)
ICSQoL	Donovan *et al* (1997)

Prevalence of lower urinary tract symptoms

Moderate to severe LUTS are relatively common, occuring in 29–51% of
a sample of 1088 men in the UK aged 50 years and over (Trueman *et al*,
1999) (see Table 1.4). However, Trueman only assessed urinary symptoms and ignored pain when he used the I-PSS as his method of assessment. Only half of the men with moderate to severe symptoms had
sought medical attention (Trueman *et al*, 1999). The main reasons given
for seeking a consultation were 'symptoms may get worse', 'fear of
cancer', 'interruption to daily activities' and 'embarrassment'.

Moderate to severe LUTS occur in about 25–30% of men aged
50 years and over who have not had surgery, and the prevalence increases
with age (Garraway *et al*, 1991; Chute *et al*, 1993; Hunter *et al*, 1996). In

Table 1.4 Age-specific prevalence of men with moderate to severe LUTS (Trueman et al, 1999 reproduced with permission)

Age group (years)	Sample n	Symptomatic n (%)
All (50–92)	1088	452 (41)
50–60	14	4 (29)
61–70	330	124 (38)
71–80	598	247 (41)
>80	146	75 (51)

the USA, the symptoms of urgency, frequency and nocturia were found to be present in 50% of men aged 62–90 years who had not undergone surgery (Milne *et al*, 1972). In the UK, the symptoms of bladder outlet obstruction most commonly due to benign prostatic hyperplasia were reported to affect 1 in 3 men over the age of 50 years (Garraway *et al*, 1991).

Summary

Male lower urinary tract symptoms (LUTS) include nocturia, frequency, urgency, urge incontinence, stress incontinence, post-micturition dribble, heistancy, weak stream, intermittency, pain, dysuria and haematuria. The IC*Smale* Questionnaire is considered to be a more accurate way than the I-PSS to assess male urinary symptoms. LUTS have a marked effect on quality of life.

CHAPTER 2

Anatomy and physiology of the male lower urinary tract

Key points

- The lower urinary tract consists of the urinary bladder and the urethra.
- The prostate gland surrounds the prostatic segment of the proximal urethra.
- The pelvic diaphragm is formed by the pubococcygeus, iliococcygeus and ischiococcygeus muscles and fasciae.
- The periurethral striated muscle consists of a mixture of fast-twitch and slow-twitch muscle fibres.

Male lower urinary tract

The lower urinary tract consists of the urinary bladder and the urethra. The proximal urethra is surrounded by the prostate gland above and the external urethral sphincter and pelvic floor muscles below.

Urinary bladder

The urinary bladder is a hollow organ located in the true pelvis (see Figure 2.1). It consists of four layers: the outer protective adventitia, the detrusor muscle, the vascular submucosa and the urothelium. The complex meshwork of smooth muscle bundles of the detrusor muscle is interspersed with collagenous supporting tissue (Gray, 1992).

Male urethra

The male urethra is between 18 cm and 20 cm long and extends from the bladder neck through the prostate and the penile shaft to its meatus at the

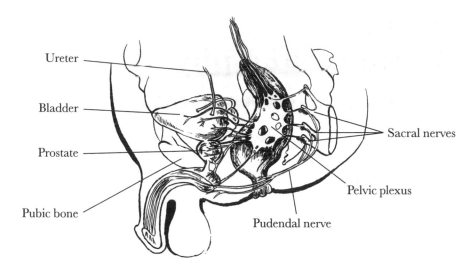

Ureter

Bladder

Prostate

Pubic bone

Sacral nerves

Pelvic plexus

Pudendal nerve

Figure 2.1 The male pelvic viscera.

glans penis, as shown in Figure 2.2. It is divided into the proximal (sphincteric) and the distal (conduit) segments. The proximal urethra is further divided into the prostatic urethra, which extends approximately 3 cm through the prostate, and the membranous urethra, which is approximately 3.5 cm long and lies just below the prostate where it pierces the pelvic floor muscles (Gray, 1992). Midway between the base and the apex of the prostate gland, the prostatic urethra angulates ventrally at about 35° (Sant and Long, 1994). The proximal urethra contains smooth muscle bundles and the specialised skeletal muscle fibres of the horseshoe-shaped external urethral sphincter (rhabdosphincter) and an inner urothelium which is lined by transitional epithelium and abundant secretory cells.

Prostate gland

The prostate gland is a small, walnut-shaped, fibromuscular gland with ducts sited at the base of the bladder surrounding the prostatic urethra as shown in Figure 2.3. The young adult prostate is about 4 cm × 3 cm × 2 cm in size and weighs about 20 g, but it gets larger with age (Neal, 1997).

The prostate gland produces fluid which provides one of the constituents of semen. The fluid contains nutrients, such as zinc (antibacterial factor) and citrate (sperm transport), enabling sperm motility and

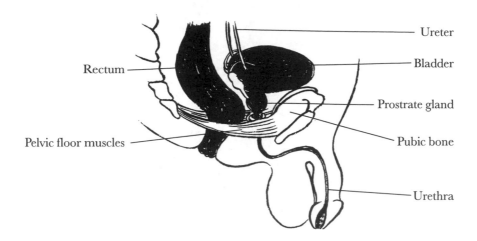

Figure 2.2 The male lower urinary tract.

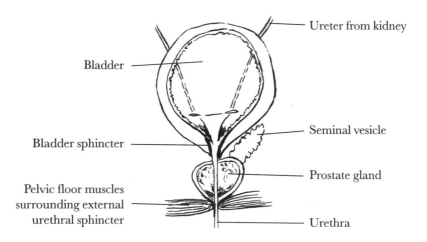

Figure 2.3 The normal bladder and prostate gland.

mobility (Sant and Long, 1994). Prostate specific antigen (PSA), a protein secreted by the prostate gland, may be found in the bloodstream. The smooth muscle of the bladder neck contracts to prevent urine escaping and semen entering the bladder during ejaculation. The prostate gland gradually enlarges with age (Figure 2.2) in the presence of androgens, especially dihydrotestosterone causing benign prostatic hyperplasia (BPH). When microscopic changes become macroscopic, symptoms of urethral obstruction may develop (Sant and Long, 1994; Neal, 1997) (see Table 2.1).

Table 2.1 The prevalence of clinical BPH and symptoms with ageing (Neal, 1997 reproduced with permission)

Age (years)	Microscopic (%)	Gross (%)	Severe symptoms (%)
35–44	8	2	0
45–54	23	8	0
55–64	42	21	2–5
65–74	71	35	8–15
75–84	82	44	15–20
>85	88	53	20–30

Pelvic floor muscles

In the male the pelvic floor muscles (PFMs) extend from the anterior to the posterior of the bony pelvis, forming a diaphragm covering the pelvic outlet which supports the urethrovesical system and rectum (see Figures 2.4 and 2.5). The puborectalis muscle forms a sling from the pubic bone round the rectum. The PFMs are divided into superior and inferior divisions. The superior portion forms part of the rectal sphincter and the periurethral muscles that contribute to the urethral sphincter mechanism. The inferior portion of the PFMs contributes primarily to the rectal gutter (Gray, 1992).

Gosling *et al* (1981) reported that the PFMs were made up of about two-thirds type 1, slow-twitch, aerobic oxidative fibres which were continuously tonic to support the pelvic viscera. The periurethral striated muscle is a mixture of fast-twitch and slow-twitch muscle fibres that raise urethral closure pressure during periods of increased intra-abdominal pressure or by voluntary control (DeLancey, 1994).

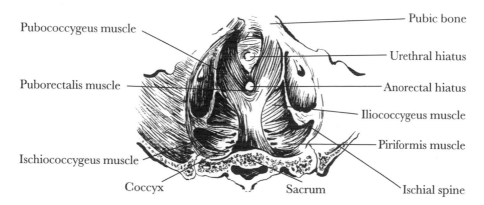

Figure 2.4 Superior view of the male pelvic floor muscles.

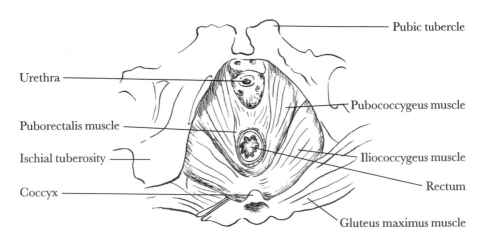

Figure 2.5 Inferior view of the male pelvic floor muscles.

Levator ani

The levator ani consists of the pubococcygeus muscle together with the iliococcygeus muscle. The pubococcygeus and iliococcygeus muscles together with the ischiococcygeus muscle form a muscular diaphragm which supports the pelvic viscera and opposes the downward thrust caused by an increase in intra-abdominal pressure.

Pubococcygeus muscle

The pubococcygeus muscle arises from the back of the pubic bone and the anterior part of the obturator fascia and inserts into a fibro-muscular layer between the anal canal and the coccyx. In animals, the pubococcygeus draws the tail under the body.

Iliococcygeus muscle

The iliococcygeus muscle arises from the ischial spine and from the tendinous arch (arcus tendineus) of the pelvic fascia and is attached to the coccyx and the median raphe. In animals, the iliococcygeus wags the tail.

Ischiococcygeus muscle

The ischiococcygeus arises from the pelvic surface of the ischial spine and is inserted into the side of the coccyx and lower sacrum. It is responsible for pulling the coccyx forward after defaecation.

Puborectalis muscle

The puborectalis muscle arises from the pelvic surface of the pubic bone, blends with the levator ani and is inserted into the muscle from the other side posterior to the rectum at the anorectal flexure. It can be considered part of the pubococcygeus muscle. It helps to maintain faecal continence by maintaining the anorectal angle.

External urethral sphincter

The intrinsic striated muscle of the external urethral sphincter mechanism in the urethra is called the rhabdosphincter (Dixon and Gosling, 1994). It surrounds the membranous urethra and lies deep to the urogenital diaphragm. It is made up of slow-twitch fibres of small diameter without muscle spindles and is postulated to receive triple innervation from the sympathetic, parasympathetic and somatic nervous systems (Gray, 1998). The superficial muscle fibres arise from the transverse perineal ligament and surrounding fascia and insert into the perineal body. The deep fibres form a continuous circular formation round the membranous urethra. The muscles from both sides together form a sphincter compressing the membranous urethra and assisting in the maintenance of urinary continence. They are relaxed during micturition and at the end of micturition, together with the bulbocavernosus muscles, they expel the last few drops of urine.

Gosling et al (1981) reported the presence of only slow-twitch fibres in the rhabdosphincter. However, in a study using histochemical techniques and electron microscopy, Light et al (1997) suggested that the rhabdosphincter consisted of two-thirds slow-twitch fibres and one-third fast-twitch fibres which enabled the sphincter to maintain urethral closure at rest and during physical activity.

Male continence mechanism

The continence mechanism in men consists of the continuous smooth muscular structure of the bladder base, the bladder neck and the proximal urethra supplemented by the striated muscle fibres of the horseshoe-shaped rhabdosphincter (Elbadawi, 1995). It was Elbadawi who led thinking away from the previous concept of a separate internal and external sphincter, describing instead a 'continuous' continence mechanism. The proportion of striated muscle cells in the rhabdosphincter decreases with age from approximately 79% in infants to 35% in an 83 year old man (Strasser et al, 1997).

Anal sphincter

The anal sphincter consists of elliptical muscle fibres each side of the anal canal attached to the tip of the coccyx posteriorly and inserted into the perineal body anteriorly. Inferiorly it blends with the skin surrounding the anus and superiorly it forms a complete sphincter and blends with the puborectalis muscle. It is normally in a state of tonic contraction but can provide greater occlusion of the anal aperture when necessary to contain faeces and flatus.

Bulbocavernosus (bulbospongiosus) muscle

The bulbocavernosous muscle, also called the bulbospongiosus muscle, arises from the median raphe and the perineal body. The middle fibres encircle the bulb and corpus spongiosum penis. The bulbocavernosus muscle empties the urethra at the end of micturition. The middle fibres assist in erection of the corpus spongiosum penis by compressing the erectile tissue of the bulb. The anterior fibres spead out over the side of the corpus cavernosum and are attached to the fascia covering the dorsal vessels of the penis. They contribute to erection by compressing the deep dorsal vein of the penis. The bulbocavernosus muscle empties the bulbar canal of the urethra. The fibres are relaxed during voiding and come into action to arrest micturition. Rhythmic contractions of the bulbocavernosus muscle propel the semen down the urethra resulting in ejaculation.

Ischiocavernosus muscle

The ischiocavernosus muscle arises from the inner surface of the ischial tuberosity and pubic ramus and inserts into an aponeurosis into the sides and undersurface of the crus penis. Contractions of the ischiocavernosus muscles produce an increase in the intracavernous pressure and influence penile rigidity (see Chapter 10, Erectile dysfunction).

Cremaster muscle

This muscle originates from the middle of the inguinal ligament where its fibres are continuous with the internal oblique muscle and occasionally with the transversus muscle. It passes anterior and lateral to the spermatic cord through the inguinal ring to insert into the cremasteric fascia surrounding the testis. The muscle fibres ascend along the medial and posterior surface of the cord and are inserted into the pubic tubercle and crest of the pubis and front of the rectus abdominis sheath. The cremaster muscle pulls the testis towards the inguinal ring during a strong contraction of the PFMs. Stroking the medial side of the thigh evokes a reflex contraction of this muscle (cremasteric reflex). The cremaster muscle is not usually under voluntary control. It is supplied by the genital branch of the genitofemoral nerve (L1 and 2).

Penis

The penis consists of three cylindrical erectile bodies: dorsally the two corpora cavernosa communicate with each other for three-quarters of their length and ventrally the corpus spongiosum surrounds the penile portion of the urethra. The proximal end of the corpus spongiosum forms a bulb attached to the urogenital diaphragm and at the distal end expands to form the glans penis (Kirby *et al*, 1999).

Nerve supply to the urinary system

The autonomic nervous system includes all efferent pathways having ganglionic synapses outside the central nervous system (Levin and Wein, 1995), and includes all smooth muscle cells. It is divided into the sympathetic and parasympathetic divisions. The sympathetic division supplying the urinary system consists of fibres originating in the thoracic and lumbar regions (T10–L2) of the spinal cord and the parasympathetic consists of fibres originating in the cranial and sacral nerves (S2–4) (see Figure 2.6). The function of the sympathetic division is to allow bladder storage. The function of the parasympathetic division is to produce a sustained bladder contraction by stimulation of the pelvic nerves.

The normal innervation of the lower urinary tract consists of three systems, which must co-ordinate for normal bladder filling and voiding: the cholinergic and adrenergic systems, and somatic nerves.

Cholinergic system controlling the bladder

The cholinergic system consists of those receptor sites in the bladder at which acetylcholine is the neurotransmitter. Cholinergic contractile receptor sites can be blocked by the muscarinic atropine.

Adrenergic system controlling the bladder and urethra

The adrenergic system consists of those receptor sites at which catecholamine is the neurotransmitter. It includes most post-ganglionic sympathetic fibres and those fibres to the smooth muscle of the lower urinary tract. Adrenergic receptors are classified either α or β. The α-adrenergic effects cause vasoconstriction and contraction of smooth muscle fibres, whereas β-adrenergic effects cause vasodilation and smooth muscle relaxation.

The bladder is innervated by the second, third and fourth sacral nerves (S2–4). The nerve supply to the external urethral sphincter is an area of debate. Studies in cats suggest that it is innervated by a combination of autonomic nerves via the pelvic plexus and somatic nerves via the pudendal nerve (Elbadawi and Schenk, 1974). Narayan *et al* (1995) demonstrated innervation by several branches from the dorsal nerve of the penis after it splits from the pudendal nerve.

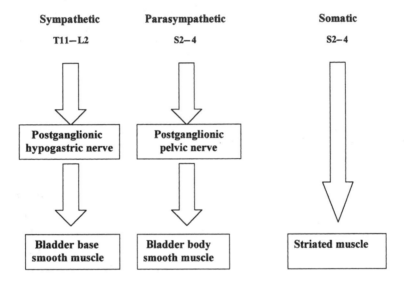

Figure 2.6 Preganglionic and postganglionic neurotransmitters.

Somatic nerves (pudendal nerves) serving the PFMs

The external anal sphincter is supplied by the perineal branch of the fourth sacral nerve and by twigs from the inferior rectal branch (S2–3) whereas the levator ani, ischiococcygeus and bulbocavernosus (bulbospongiosus) are supplied by the perineal branch of the pudendal nerve (S2–4).

Sacral dermatomes

The dermatome from the second sacral nerve (S2) extends over the lateral aspect of the buttocks and thigh and the posterior aspect of the calf and plantar surface of the heel. The dermatome from the third sacral nerve (S3) covers an area over the upper two-thirds of the medial aspect of the thigh. The dermatome from the fourth sacral nerve (S4) extends over the penis and perineal area (see Figure 2.7).

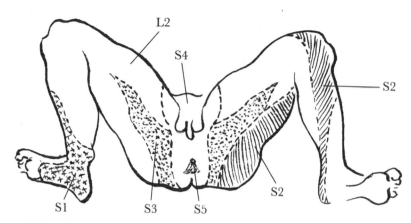

Figure 2.7 Sacral dermatomes.

Congenital abnormalities

Hypospadias

Hypospadias (Figure 2.8) is a congenital abnormality where the urethral meatus opens on the underside (ventral surface) of the penis anywhere along the penis from the meatus to the scotum. It may be associated with chordee, where the glans penis bends ventrally and the penis has a ventral angulation. It is usually repaired in the young by surgery.

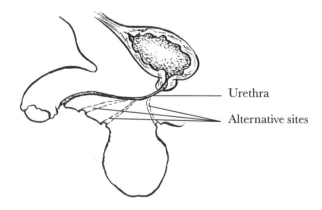

Figure 2.8 Hypospadias.

Epispadias

Epispadias (Figure 2.9) is a rarer congenital abnormality where the urethral meatus opens at an abnormal position on the upper (dorsal surface) of the penis. It too is usually repaired in the young by surgery.

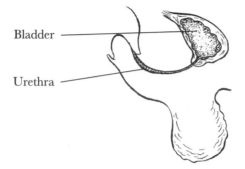

Figure 2.9 Epispadias.

Urethral and ureteral valves

Occasionally, boys may be born with urethral valves caused by an abnormal fold of the urethra in the prostatic, membranous or proximal bulbar section (Caldamone, 1994), or with malformed and incompetent ureteral valves at the junction of the ureter and bladder. These valves cause reflux of urine, with the danger of hydronephrosis and ultimately renal failure. Early surgical intervention is paramount.

Exstrophy of the bladder

A serious congenital abnormality occurs when the abdominal wall fails to develop and the bladder fails to close, leaving the ureters on the surface of the abdomen and the bladder exposed (Caldamone, 1994) (Figure 2.10).

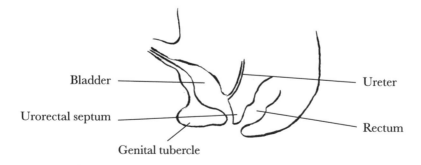

Figure 2.10 Exstrophy of the bladder.

The bladder has to be reconstructed surgically or the ureters diverted to form an ileal conduit (opening of the ureters through the abdominal wall using a portion of the ileum).

Ureteral ectopia

An ectopic ureter has its insertion directly into the urethra instead of into the trigone area of the bladder. If the insertion level is below the external urethral sphincter, it may cause continuous incontinence. It is sometimes associated with duplex ureters. Ureteral ectopia is repaired by surgery.

Primary obstructive megaureter

A primary obstructive megaureter occurs as a result of a derangement of the ureteral musculature which impedes the normal peristalsis conveying a bolus of urine (Caldamone, 1994). A developmental arrest of the longitudinal musculature may lead to a non-peristaltic segment of ureter, causing obstruction.

Secondary obstructive megaureter

An incompetent ureteral valve at the lower end of the ureter as it passes through the bladder wall may cause secondary reflux and a megaureter (Figure 2.11).

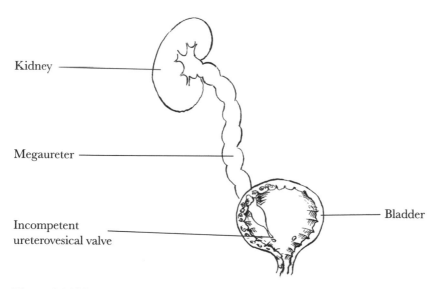

Kidney

Megaureter

Incompetent
ureterovesical valve

Bladder

Figure 2.11 Megaureter.

Summary

The lower urinary tract consists of the urinary bladder and the urethra. The prostate gland surrounds the prostatic segment of the proximal urethra. The pelvic diaphragm is formed by the pubococcygeus, iliococcygeus and ischiococcygeus muscles and fasciae. Congenital abnormalities may affect any part of the urinary system.

CHAPTER 3

Urinary continence

Key points

- The continence mechanism in men consists of the bladder base, the bladder neck and the proximal urethra supplemented by the rhabdosphincter.
- Urinary continence relies on an intact urinary system, integration of the brain, spinal cord, peripheral nervous system and a competent urethral sphincter.
- Neurological integral reflexes control normal bladder storage and voiding.

Urinary continence relies on three mechanisms: an anatomically intact urinary system; integration of neural modulatory structures in the brain, spinal cord and peripheral nervous system; and a competent urethral sphincter mechanism (Gray, 1992; Park *et al*, 1997). Maintenance of urinary continence is multifactorial and depends on detrusor control and urethral closure function (Bernstein, 1997). Passive urethral closure is enhanced by the activity of the rhabdosphincter muscle and the use of the PFMs, particularly in the presence of increased intra-abdominal pressure.

Micturition cycle

Filling phase

The urine produced by the kidneys is propelled along the ureters into the bladder by peristalsis activity of the smooth ureteric muscle. The visco-elastic bladder is compliant to the volume of urine produced so that the bladder pressure remains at zero. When the bladder fills to 350–500 ml, the intravesical stretch receptors are stimulated via S2–4 which trigger a detrusor muscle contraction and a strong desire to void. The first sensation of filling is usually at approximately 200 ml. This initial desire to void can be normally controlled and voiding will usually take place following a strong desire to void (see Figure 3.1).

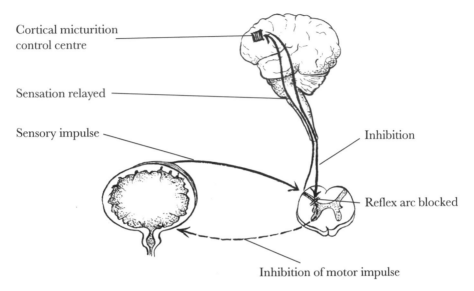

Cortical micturition control centre

Sensation relayed

Sensory impulse

Inhibition

Reflex arc blocked

Inhibition of motor impulse

Figure 3.1 Bladder filling.

Voiding phase

Voiding is initiated by the relaxation of the striated musculature under voluntary control and voiding is completed by reflex action. The detrusor muscle contracts increasing the internal pressure in the bladder. Urine passes through the relaxed involuntary and voluntary muscle of the urethra. Voiding occurs at approximately 15 ml/s in a male (20 ml/s in the female), although it is faster in the young. In normal men maximum flow rates are obtained at volumes of 300–400 ml, and flow rate is improved by a standing position (Berger, 1995). Normally the bladder empties completely (see Figure 3.2).

Refilling phase

After micturition, the external urethral muscles and the PFMs including the bulbocavernosus muscles contract while the detrusor muscle relaxes enabling the bladder to refill, thus repeating the micturition cycle.

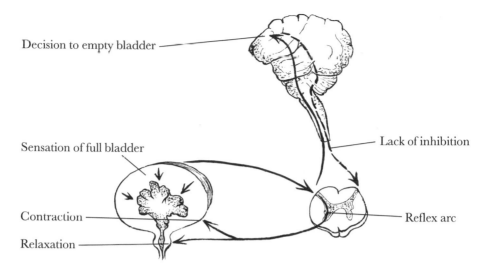

Figure 3.2 Bladder voiding.

Neurological control of the bladder

The neurological control of the bladder is a complex subject and the local interactions between neurological modulators of the urethra and detrusor are not altogether clear (Gray, 1996).

The detrusor muscle is under neurological control from the brain, the spinal cord, the peripheral nerves and the neurotransmitters of the lower urinary tract (Gray, 1998) (see Figure 3.3).

Brain

The frontal lobes of the cerebral cortex contain a detrusor motor area (Andrew *et al*, 1964). The thalamus may have an inhibitory effect on detrusor contractility (Gray, 1998). The basal ganglia exert an inhibitory influence on the detrusor reflex, allowing continence control. The hypothalamus may exert some influence but its function is unclear (Torrens, 1987). The pontine micturition centre activates detrusor contraction and sphincteric co-ordination (Griffiths *et al*, 1990). In infants micturition is a pontine reflex (Gray, 1996).

Spinal cord

The spinal cord influences lower urinary tract function (Gray, 1996). There is still controversy about the role of the sacral micturition reflex centre (SMRC). However, the sacral reflex is mediated by the pelvic and pudendal nerves and is subject to facilitation or inhibition by descending central nervous system pathways (Levin and Wein, 1995).

Sympathetic control

Bladder storage is under sympathetic control. Sympathetic stimulation of the bladder promotes detrusor relaxation and bladder filling via the afferent and efferent tracts arising between T10 and L2 spinal segments. The inferior hypogastric plexus provides sympathetic input for the detrusor muscle.

Parasympathetic control

Voiding is under parasympathetic control. Parasympathetic stimulation produces a detrusor contraction and urethral sphincter relaxation via the afferent and efferent tracts located in S2–4 pelvic plexus.

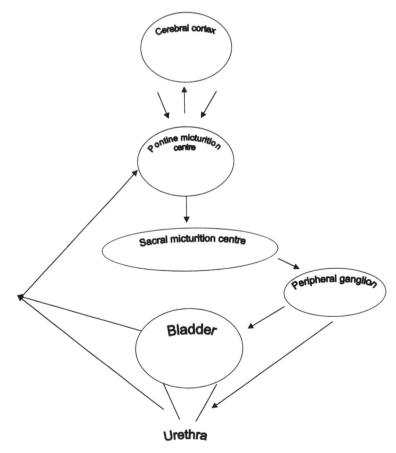

Figure 3.3 Neurological control of the bladder.

Peripheral nerves

The bladder is innervated by the pelvic nerve arising from the second, third and fourth sacral nerves (S2–4). The levator ani, ischicoccygeus and bulbocavernosus are supplied by the perineal branch of the pudendal nerve (S2–4). The nerve supply to the external urethral sphincter is from the pudendal nerve (S2–4). The periurethral muscle receives innervation from the pudendal nerve (S1–3) (Gray, 1998).

Neurotransmitters

The detrusor muscle is a smooth muscle which contains actin and myosin filaments. It relies on calcium ions to contract (Steers, 1992). The primary neurotransmitter acetylcholine is released under parasympathetic control causing a detrusor contraction and voiding, whereas noradrenaline under control of the sympathetic system is the primary neurotransmitter causing inhibition of the detrusor muscle and allowing storage to take place.

Integral bladder storage and voiding reflexes

Mahony *et al* (1977) described neurological integral reflexes which control bladder storage and voiding. Overactivity or functional failure of one or more integral reflexes may cause a significant disorder of lower urinary tract function.

Bladder storage reflexes

Sympathetic stimulation causes bladder relaxation and contraction of the bladder neck (Mahony *et al*, 1977). In response to increased tension in the bladder wall, there is relaxation of the detrusor muscle and contraction of the internal and external urethral sphincters by the sympathetic detrusor inhibiting reflex (SDIR) and the sympathetic sphincter-constrictor reflex (SSCR). The perineodetrusor inhibitory reflex (PDIR) produces a further relaxation of the detrusor muscle in response to an increase in pelvic floor muscle tone causing an inhibitory influence on the sacral micturition centre. Feedback concerning the resting tone of the PFMs and the external urethral sphincter is provided by the perineopudendal facilitative reflex (PPFR). If there is an increase in trigonal and bladder neck pressure or if urine escapes into the proximal urethra, a urethrosphincteric guarding reflex (USGR) causes an increase in tone in the external urethral sphincter. Somatic stimulation causes contraction of the external sphincter of the urethra. Two descending pathways from higher centres control and inhibit the autonomic sacral voiding reflex and relaxes this inhibition when appropriate (see Table 3.1).

Bladder voiding reflexes

Parasympathetic stimulation causes contraction of the detrusor muscle and relaxation of the internal urethral sphincter (Mahony *et al*, 1977). Voluntary contractions of the abdominal muscles and the diaphragm and simultaneous relaxation of the PFMs facilitate micturition via the perineobulbar detrusor facilitative reflex (PBDFR). Increased pressure to the detrusor facilitates the detrusodetrusor facilitative reflex (DDFR) to initiate voluntary micturition. Once initiated, voiding is continued by control of the detrusourethral inhibitory reflex (DUIR) which results in inhibition of the bladder neck and the proximal urethra in response to the detrusor mural pressure. The detrusosphincteric inhibitory reflex (DSIR) results in inhibition of the sphincter in response to increased detrusor pressure. Urine in the urethra stimulates the continuation of detrusor contraction and sphincter relaxation via the urethrodetrusor facilitative reflex

Table 3.1 Bladder storage reflexes (Mahony *et al*, 1977)

Reflex	Trigger	Effect	Afferent nerve	Efferent nerve
SDIR	Detrusor mural (wall) pressure increase	Detrusor relaxation	Pelvic nerve via thoracolumbar cord	Hypogastric nerve
SSCR	Detrusor mural pressure increase	Internal sphincter contraction	Pelvic nerve via thoracolumbar cord	Hypogastric nerve
PDIR	Increased PFM tone	Detrusor relaxation	Pudendal nerve via sacral micturition reflex centre	Pelvic nerve
PPFR	Detrusor mural pressure increase	PFM and external urethral sphincter resting tone	Pudendal nerve via sacral micturition reflex centre	Pudendal nerve
USGR	Trigonal and bladder neck pressure increase Urine in proximal urethra	Increased tone in external urethral sphincter	Pudendal nerve via pudendal nucleus in spinal cord	Pudendal nerve

(UDFR) and the urethrosphincteric inhibitory reflex (USIR). The voluntary contraction of the PFMs inhibits the action of the detrusor muscle via the perineobulbar detrusor inhibitory reflex (PBDIR); voiding ceases, and there is a return to the storage phase (see Table 3.2).

Table 3.2 Bladder voiding reflexes (Mahony *et al*, 1977)

Reflex	Trigger	Effect	Afferent nerve	Efferent nerve
PBDFR	Contraction of abdominals and diaphragm and relaxation of pelvic floor muscles	Initiate micturition	Pudendal nerve to sacrobulbar tract via medulla and SMRC	Hypogastric nerve
DDFR	Detrusor mural pressure increase	Initiate micturition	Pudendal nerve and lateral funiculus via pons and sacral micturition reflex centre	Lateral reticulospinal tract and pelvic nerve
DUIR	Detrusor mural pressure increase	Bladder neck and proximal urethra relaxation	Pelvic nerve via sacral micturition reflex centre	Pelvic nerve
DSIR	Detrusor mural pressure increase	External urethral sphincter relaxation	Pelvic nerve via pudendal nucleus sacral cord	Pudendal nerve
UDFR	Urine in urethra	Detrusor contraction and external urethral sphincter relaxation	Pelvic nerve and dorsal funiculus via pons and sacral micturition reflex centre	Lateral reticulospinal tract and pelvic nerve
USIR	Urine flow across urethral mucosa	External urethral sphincter relaxation	Pudendal nerve via pudendal nucleus sacral cord	Pudendal nerve
PBDIR	Contraction of pelvic floor muscles	Cessation of voiding	Pudendal nerve and sacrobulbar tract via medulla and SMRC	Ventral reticulospinal tract

Summary

The continence mechanism in men consists of the bladder base, the bladder neck and the proximal urethra supplemented by the rhabdosphincter. Urinary continence relies on an intact urinary system, integration of the brain, spinal cord, peripheral nervous system and a competent urethral sphincter.

Micturition reflexes can be subdivided into four groups depending on the stage of the micturition cycle:

1. Reflexes concerned with storage;
2. Reflexes concerned with preparation to void;
3. Reflexes allowing voiding to continue;
4. Reflexes concerned with preparation to store.

CHAPTER 4

Prostate conditions and their treatment

Key points

- The most common prostate conditions are benign prostatic hyperplasia (BPH), prostate cancer and prostatitis.
- The prevalence of BPH increases with age.
- Prostate cancer accounts for 1 in 10 deaths in Europe and North America.
- There are four types of prostatitis: acute bacterial, chronic bacterial, non-bacterial (prostatosis) and prostatodynia.

Investigations for prostate conditions

Tests which assist in the diagnosis of BPH and prostate cancer are:

- Urinalysis of mid-stream urine to eliminate urinary infection.
- Uroflow, to assess the flow rate during micturition. A reduced flow rate and a high residual volume of urine in the bladder may demonstrate blockage (see Figure 4.1).
- Estimation of volume of urine after voiding using ultrasound over the lower abdomen to test for retention of urine in the bladder.
- Digital rectal examination (DRE), in side-lying or forward bending to assess size and consistency of the prostate gland. Abnormal irregularities may be indicative of prostate cancer.
- Prostate specific antigen (PSA) blood test in men between 50 and 75 years of age. This is not definitive but is used in conjunction with other tests.
- Rectal ultrasound scan to aid the diagnosis of prostatic cancer and BPH.
- Urodynamics to diagnose sphincter/bladder dysfunction.

- Flexible cystoscopy for the diagnosis of strictures, interstitial cystitis and bladder tumours
- Radiography of kidneys, ureters and bladder (KUB) for stones, bladder tumours and foreign bodies
- Intravenous pyelogram (IVP) to assess upper urinary tract problems
- Cystogram to aid the diagnosis of bladder pathology
- F/V chart to monitor amount and timing of fluid input and output.

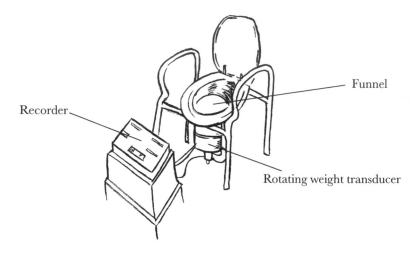

Figure 4.1 Uroflowmeter.

Benign prostatic hyperplasia

BPH is a condition which includes benign prostatic enlargement (BPE) due to a multiplication of normal cells, lower urinary tract symptoms (LUTS) and bladder outlet obstruction (BOO). The prevalence of BPE increases with age. In a study of 597 men by Simpson *et al* (1996), the age-specific rates for BPE, using the threshold of a prostate size of over 20 g, was reported to be 62% for men 40–49 years of age, 78% for men 50–59 years of age, 89% for men 60–69 years of age and 89% for men 70–79 years of age. However, they found no significant relationship between prostate size and symptoms.

Pathologic BPH is divided into two stages: microscopic and macroscopic (Sant and Long, 1994). The earliest microscopic nodules of BPH develop in men between 30 and 50 years of age in the periurethral zone and may infiltrate the transitional zone. The aetiology of BPH is imprecisely defined. Ageing and the presence of androgens, especially dihydrotestosterone, are essential factors for the development of BPH.

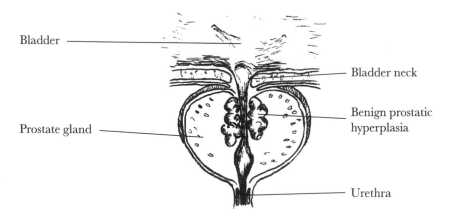

Bladder

Bladder neck

Benign prostatic
hyperplasia

Prostate gland

Urethra

Figure 4.2 Benign prostatic hyperplasia.

Treatment for BPH

Transurethral resection of prostate (TURP) is the most frequently
performed operation for BPH and is performed using a resectoscope with
a cutting loop and coagulating electrode. In all forms of prostatectomy,
the bladder neck is resected rendering the closure mechanism incompetent. Postoperative continence relies on the strength and integrity of the
external urinary sphincter. Men may experience retrograde ejaculation
after prostatectomy. During normal ejaculation, closure of the bladder neck
prevents seminal fluid entering the bladder. However, after surgery the
seminal fluid may enter the bladder and is voided at the next micturition.

A retropubic or suprapubic prostatectomy is occasionally performed
for larger prostates with BPH. Surgery is performed through a lower
abdominal incision. The prostate gland is surgically enucleated leaving
the outer capsule intact.

The range of minimally invasive treatments for men with BPH has
grown steadily in the last decade. The energy sources range from
microwaves and radiofrequency waves to high intensity focused ultrasound, laser vaporisation/coagulation/resection and electrosurgical
techniques (Djavan *et al*, 1999). However, TURP is still considered the
gold standard. A systematic review of six studies comparing laser surgery
to TURP was unable to make a definitive judgement about safety, efficacy and durability because of the poor methodology of the studies
(Wheelahan *et al*, 2000).

As an alternative to surgery, other treatments such as drug therapy or
stents may be advised. Patients will be guided by their urologist to make

an informed choice from the different treatments available. Two drug therapy treatments are available for the reduction of urinary symptoms caused by benign prostatic enlargement (see Chapter 9). For men with retention but who are unfit for surgery, wire or silicone mesh stents may be positioned inside the restricted prostatic urethra to allow the free flow of urine. Unfortunately, various problems can arise with the use of stents. They can cause infection and are prone to encrustation or even migration into the bladder.

Prostate cancer

In the UK prostate cancer is the fourth commonest cancer in men, after skin, lung and large bowel cancer (Chamberlain *et al* (1997), and in Europe and North America it is the second most lethal malignancy after lung cancer. In England and Wales the incidence is 54.2 per 100 000 of population in males of all ages (Chamberlain *et al*, 1997), accounting for 1 in 10 deaths in Europe and North America (Kirby *et al*, 1994). In the UK it accounts for 8848 deaths a year (OPCS, 1996). In the majority of cases prostate cancer occurs as the result of primary tumours (Gray, 1992). Cancer is caused by a multiplication of abnormal cells and is associated with loss of apoptotic potential (where cells lose the ability to die) and uncontrolled proliferation (where cells proliferate out of control) (Denmeade *et al*, 1996). Prostate adenocarcinomas originate within the stroma (cortex) of the gland with a firm, single or multifocal nodule. As the tumour volume increases, it causes enlargement of the prostate gland, which may give rise to symptoms of bladder outlet obstruction. The cause of prostate adenocarcinoma remains unclear but genetic, racial, viral and dietary factors have been suggested.

BPH and prostate cancer are two separate entities. One does not lead to the other, but they may co-exist. Prostate cancer may be slowly growing in the elderly, who may die 'with' rather than 'of' the disease.

Treatment of prostate cancer

For prostate cancer, patients may be given the choice of a radical prostatectomy, radiotherapy (called brachytherapy if radioactive seeds are used), anti-androgen treatment or more rarely now orchidectomy. Shared decision-making is now considered to be an integral part of gaining informed consent from patients for most urological surgery. Emberton *et al* (1997) have produced an interactive CD-ROM multimedia patient information package for men with LUTS which can be used to aid decision-making. Radical prostatectomy is becoming increasingly preferred

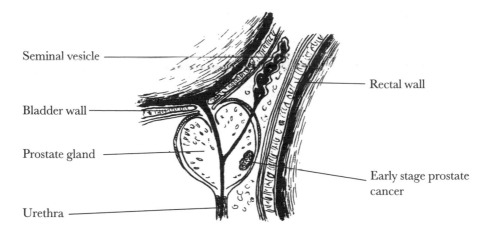

Seminal vesicle

Rectal wall

Bladder wall

Prostate gland

Early stage prostate cancer

Urethra

Figure 4.3 Prostate cancer.

for localised disease, particularly now that nerve sparing techniques can help to preserve potency and continence (Resnick, 1992).

Urethral stricture

Urethral stricture occurs when scar tissue narrows the urethra following urethritis (infection of the urethra) or trauma. It may occur at any part of the urethra from the meatus (external opening) to the prostatic urethra. At the peno-scrotal junction, strictures form from traumatic catheterisation (Denning, 1996).

Treatment of a stricture consists of dilatation under anaesthetic or surgical division by urethrotomy. Maintenance treatment may consist of regular dilatation by intermittent self-catheterisation (ISC) (Lawrence and MacDonagh, 1988).

Sphincterotomy

A sphincterotomy is an operation where the proximal sphincter at the bladder neck or the external urinary sphincter is cut to allow the passage of urine. Blockage is due to spasm of the sphincter, which occurs during detrusor/sphincter dyssynergia.

Prostatitis

There are four types of prostatitis: acute bacterial, chronic bacterial, non-bacterial (prostatosis) and prostatodynia. Each type may cause considerable rectal and suprapubic discomfort (see Chapter 6).

Summary

There are a number of investigations which may assist in the diagnosis of BPH, prostate cancer and prostatitis. These three separate prostate conditions may co-exist. There are a number of treatment options for each condition.

CHAPTER 5

Urinary incontinence

Key points

- Urinary incontinence is defined as the involuntary loss of urine which is objectively demonstrable and a social or hygienic problem.
- There are a number of classification systems for different types of incontinence.
- The prevalence of urinary incontinence ranges from 3.6% in men 45 years old to 28.2% in men 90 years old.

Definition

Urinary incontinence is defined by the International Continence Society (ICS) as 'the involuntary loss of urine which is objectively demonstrable and a social or hygienic problem' (Abrams *et al*, 1998b). The condition of urinary incontinence is defined as the pathophysiology underlying incontinence, as demonstrated by clinical or urodynamic techniques (Blaivas *et al*, 1997).

Prevalence of urinary incontinence in men

The absolute incidence of urinary incontinence among men in the UK remains unknown. Urinary incontinence is an under-reported problem, probably because of the social stigma (Gray, 1992). Patients may be too embarrassed to consult their doctor. Perhaps all patients should be questioned tactfully about their continence status when presenting to any medical professional. Many cases of urinary incontinence are transient, brought on by infection, immobility or acute disease. However, many others represent a chronic condition that persists until proper treatment and bladder management strategies allowing social continence are instituted (Gray, 1992).

The prevalence of urinary incontinence in men increases with age and ranges from 3.6% in men 45 years old to 28.2% in men 90 years old or older (Thomas *et al*, 1980; Britton *et al*, 1990; Brocklehurst, 1993; Malmsten *et al*, 1997). The prevalence of reported urinary incontinence in men also varies with the definition of incontinence and the threshold of incontinence used. In many of the larger studies incontinence was defined in different ways, making a true comparison impossible. For example, Britton *et al* (1990) found an incidence of 27% in 578 men aged 60–85 years of age who attended a screening clinic in Leeds and completed a self-administered questionnaire. Incontinence was defined as 'Dribbling into pants at any time'. Brocklehurst (1993) interviewed a random sample of 4007 community-dwelling adults, of whom, 1883 were men aged 30 and over, and used the definition of urinary incontinence as 'Any leaking, wet pants or damp pants?' and the threshold of 'Have you ever suffered from?'. The study revealed 6.6% (124 men) had been incontinent of urine at some time. Of these, 60% (74 men) were worried or concerned about their incontinence and almost 50% experienced limitation of daily activities such as using public transport, visiting friends and going to work.

Incidence of urinary incontinence following transurethral resection of the prostate

TURP is one of the most frequently performed surgical procedures in the UK, with about 20% of men over 50 years likely to undergo resection (Garraway *et al*, 1991). Every year about 50 000 men in Great Britain have prostate surgery (Office of Health Economics, 1995). A survey in England of 5276 patients who had undergone TURP found that a third (1759 men) who were continent before surgery reported some incontinence 3 months after prostatectomy (Emberton *et al*, 1996). In a confidential questionnaire by the Royal College of Surgeons in England as part of the National Prostatectomy Audit, 6% of patients who stated they were continent before TURP described severe incontinence or the use of pads 3 months after operation (Neal, 1997).

Incidence of urinary incontinence following radical prostatectomy

Donnellan *et al* (1997) reported 6% mildly incontinent, 6% moderately incontinent and 4% severely incontinent at 1 year after radical prostatectomy. No patient reported preoperative incontinence, but after surgery urinary incontinence was reported to be the most distressing problem. Davidson *et al* (1996) investigated 188 previously continent men following radical prostatectomy. They graded incontinence as grade 1 (patients needing 1–2 pads per day) and grade 2 (patients who needed 2 or more pads per day). They found that the amount of the initial loss did not predict the time to continence. The results for both grades combined showed that 107 (56%) were incontinent postoperatively after catheter removal, 40 (21%) were incontinent at 3 months and 24 (14%) were still incontinent at 1 year. However, Rudy *et al* (1984) reported incontinence following radical prostatectomy to be as high as 87% at 6 months after surgery, on the basis of strict urodynamic testing criteria. The definition of incontinence used was 'the occasional pad'. This paper was written before the introduction of nerve sparing surgery.

Koeman *et al* (1996) used a self-administered questionnaire and reported that after radical prostatectomy 9 out of 14 men had involuntary loss of urine at orgasm, even though only one patient suffered from stress incontinence. Koeman *et al* (1996) reported that the prevalence of this type of leakage may be higher than previously thought. Moul (1994) and Paulson (1991) both state that incontinence after prostatectomy may be avoided by adhering to careful surgical technique.

Classification of incontinence

Incontinence may be classified into stress incontinence, urge incontinence, mixed incontinence, post-micturition dribble, reflex incontinence, overflow incontinence, extra-urethral incontinence and functional incontinence.

Stress incontinence

Stress incontinence is defined as 'the complaint of involuntary loss of urine during coughing, sneezing, or physical exertion such as sport activities, sudden changes of position, etc.' (Blaivas *et al*, 1997). The ICS definition is 'the involuntary loss of urine that occurs when the intravesical pressure exceeds the maximal urethral pressure in the absence of a detrusor contraction'(Blaivas *et al*, 1997). Stress incontinence is almost always iatrogenic. Men are at risk after radical prostatectomy, radiotherapy and occasionally TURP (Figure 5.1).

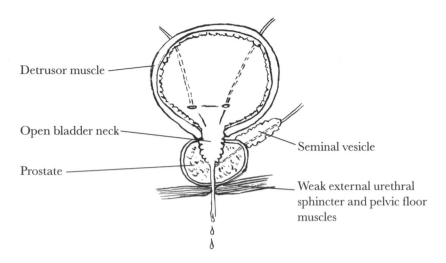

Detrusor muscle

Open bladder neck

Prostate

Seminal vesicle

Weak external urethral
sphincter and pelvic floor
muscles

Figure 5.1 Stress incontinence following transurethral resection of prostate.

Urge incontinence

The symptom urge incontinence is 'the complaint of the involuntary loss
of urine associated with a sudden, strong desire to void (urgency)' (Blaivas
et al, 1997). Urge incontinence may be caused by detrusor overactivity
(overactive bladder), detrusor instability or detrusor hyperreflexia (see
Figure 5.2).

Urgency

Urgency may be associated with two types of dysfunction; motor urgency
indicating overactive detrusor function and sensory urgency indicating
hypersensitivity of the bladder to filling (Abrams *et al*, 1998b).

Motor urgency

Motor urgency indicates overactive detrusor function (Abrams *et al*,
1998b. The condition is called detrusor instability if it is confirmed with
urodynamics, provided there is no neurological deficit.

Sensory urgency

Sensory urgency is urgency and sometimes involuntary loss of urine associated with a strong desire to void which is not due to uninhibited detrusor contractions. It has been called a hypersensitive dysfunction (Abrams
et al, 1998b).

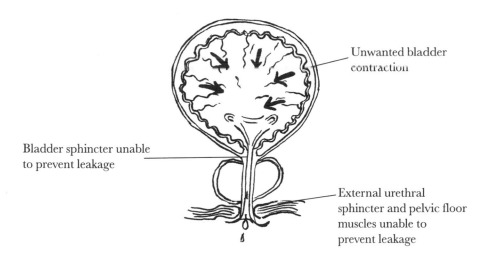

Unwanted bladder contraction

Bladder sphincter unable to prevent leakage

External urethral sphincter and pelvic floor muscles unable to prevent leakage

Figure 5.2 Urge incontinence.

Mixed incontinence

The ICS definition of mixed incontinence is 'incontinence that is a mixture of both stress and urge incontinence' (Abrams *et al*, 1998b).

Detrusor overactivity

Detrusor overactivity is the generic term for involuntary detrusor contractions. This term should be used when the aetiology of the involuntary detrusor contractions is unclear (Blaivas *et al*, 1997).

Detrusor instability

Detrusor instability denotes detrusor contractions which are not due to neurological disorders (Blaivas *et al*, 1997).

Detrusor hyperreflexia

Detrusor hyperreflexia denotes detrusor contractions which are due to neurological conditions (Blaivas *et al*, 1997).

Nocturia

Nocturia means waking at night to void urine. It can be regarded as a symptom, a condition or a feature of nocturnal polyuria (Van Kerrebroeck and Weiss, 1999). It can be assessed using the nocturia index and dividing the nightly voided urine volume by the functional bladder capacity (see Table 5.1).

The key factors associated with nocturia are summarised in Table 5.2.

Table 5.1 Definitions of the classification and aetiology of nocturia (Van Kerrebroeck and Weiss, 1999 reproduced with permission)

Variable	Definition
Nocturnal urine volume (NUV)	Nightly voided volume plus first morning voided volume
Functional bladder capacity (FBC)	Largest single recorded voided volume from 24 h voiding diary
Nocturia index (NI)	NUV/FBC
Actual number of nightly voids (ANV)	Recorded from bladder diary
Predicted number of nightly voids (PNV)	NI minus 1 (rounded to next highest integer if this is not a whole number)
Nocturnal bladder capacity index (NBCI)	ANV minus PNV; if PNV>ANV then NBCI= 0
Nocturnal polyuria index (NPI)	NUV/24 h total voided volume (normal <35%)

Table 5.2 Major factors associated with nocturia (Fonda, 1999 reproduced with permission)

Ageing
Psychogenic
Behavioural
Sleep changes, disturbance and amount of time spent in bed
Polyuria syndromes
Bladder problems
Neurological causes
Combinations of all of the above

Nocturnal polyuria

One definition of nocturnal polyuria is that the nocturnal output of urine is over 35% of the total 24 h urine production (Weiss *et al*, 1998). Nocturia increases with advancing age. By the eighth decade 80% of men get up at least once a night to void (Middlekoop *et al*, 1996). However, there are many reasons for nocturnal polyuria (see Table 5.3). Nocturnal polyuria can be assessed using the nocturnal polyuria index (NPI) and dividing the nocturnal urine volume (NUV) by the 24 h total voided urine volume (see Table 5.1).

Table 5.3 Causes of nocturnal polyuria (Van Kerrebroeck and Weiss, 1999 reproduced with permission)

Cause	Reason
Reverse nocturnal/diurnal urine production	Absence of circadian rhythmicity in arginine vasopressin (AVP) secretion: solute diuresis mediated by increased atrial natriuretic peptide (ANP) levels in patients with sleep apnoea
Polydipsia (excessive thirst)	Polyuria
	Diabetes mellitus / insipidus
	Excessive fluid intake, especially in the evening
Third-space fluid loss	Congestive heart failure
	Venous insufficiency
	Excessive salt intake
	Hypoalbumenaemia / nephrotic syndrome
Other	Late evening administration of drinks

Nocturnal enuresis

The symptom of nocturnal enuresis is the complaint of urinary loss which occurs only during sleep (Blaivas *et al*, 1997). The cause remains obscure. Hereditary factors, sleep disturbance and natriuresis (excretion of sodium ions) may play a part, but remain unproven. In children enuresis may be caused by incomplete bladder emptying. There are similarities between enuresis and nocturia where both entities are based on nocturnal polyuria with urine production exceeding the bladder capacity. The absence of a circadian rhythm in arginine vasopressin (AVP) is also associated with both enuresis and nocturia (Djurhuus *et al*, 1999).

Post-micturition dribble

Post-micturition dribble (PMD), also called post-void dribble, is the complaint of a dribbling loss of urine which occurs after voiding (Blaivas *et al*, 1997). It should be distinguished from terminal dribble which occurs at the end of micturition. The amount can be as much as 15 ml (an egg-cup full). It is a common problem for men of all ages (Pomfret, 1993), but particularly troublesome in older men (Paterson *et al*, 1997). PMD is attributed to a failure of the bulbocavernosus (bulbospongiosus) muscle to evacuate the bulbar portion of the urethra (Feneley, 1986; Millard, 1989) causing pooling of urine in the bulbar urethra which can dribble with movement. Men who suffer from PMD may prefer to wear pads or dribble collectors, but an alternative treatment is bulbar urethral massage

(Millard, 1989; Pomfret, 1993) and pelvic floor muscle exercises (Paterson *et al*, 1997) (see Chapter 8).

Reflex incontinence

Reflex incontinence is loss of urine due to detrusor hyperreflexia and/or involuntary urethral relaxation in the absence of the sensation usually associated with the desire to micturate. This condition is only seen in patients with neuropathic disorders of the bladder or urethra (Abrams *et al*, 1998b).

Overflow incontinence

Overflow incontinence is any involuntary loss of urine associated with over-distention of the bladder (Abrams *et al*, 1998b). This may be caused by obstruction, a loss of detrusor activity (atonic bladder) or impaired contractility (hypotonic bladder) due to detrusor underactivity.

Unconscious incontinence

Unconscious incontinence may occur in the absence of urge and without conscious recognition of the urinary loss (Abrams *et al*, 1998b).

Extra-urethral incontinence

Extra-urethral incontinence occurs rarely, when leakage occurs as a result of an ectopic ureter or from a fistula.

Functional incontinence

Functional incontinence occurs when men are unable to get to the bathroom in time as a result of mobility and dexterity problems.

Classification systems for urinary incontinence

There are different systems for the classification of incontinence, all of which include stress and urge incontinence, as shown in Table 5.4. However, there is controversy over some types of incontinence, especially functional incontinence. Functional problems frequently mask the real cause of the incontinence, or, conversely, functional incontinence may be caused by an inability to reach the toilet in time. This can be a most distressing problem for the elderly and immobile who would be continent without their handicap. The Urodynamic Classification includes overflow incontinence and extra-urethral incontinence under the heading 'unconscious incontinence' (Blaivas *et al*, 1997). It may be easier to keep these two categories separate.

Table 5.4 Classification systems for urinary incontinence

Gray and Doughty (1987)	North American Nursing Diagnosis Association (Barret and Wein, 1991)	Urodynamic classification (Blaivas et al, 1997)	Delphi study (Dorey, 2000f)
Instability incontinence	Urge incontinence Reflex incontinence	Urge incontinence due to detrusor overactivity	Urge incontinence due to detrusor instability and detrusor hyperreflexia
Stress incontinence	Stress incontinence	Stress incontinence due to sphincter abnormalities Unconscious incontinence due to detrusor overactivity, sphincter abnormalities, overflow or extra-urethral incontinence	Stress incontinence due to incompetent sphincter
	Total incontinence (severe sphincter incompetence)	Continuous leakage due to sphincter abnormalities or extra-urethral incontinence	Extra-urethral incontinence from urinary fistula or ectopic ureter
Overflow incontinence (urinary retention)	Urinary retention		Overflow incontinence due to BOO, acontractile bladder, detrusor/ sphincter dyssynergia
		Nocturnal enuresis due to sphincter abnormality or extra-urethral incontinence	
		Post-void dribble due to urine retained in distal urethra	Post-void dribble due to urine in bulbar urethra
All leakage with functional aspects	Functional incontinence		Functional incontinence

Summary

There are a number of different types and classifications of incontinence in men. The most common types of incontinence are stress incontinence, urge incontinence and PMD.

CHAPTER 6

Pelvic pain

Key points

- Pain syndromes of the urogenital and rectal area include orchialgia, penile pain, prostate pain and perineal pain.
- Some pain relief can be provided using pain medications, local treatment regimens, physiotherapy and psychological interventions.
- In the later stages of prostate cancer, symptoms of hip, leg and back pain may be mistaken for arthritis.

Pain syndromes of the urogenital area are well described but under-recognised and poorly understood (Wesselmann *et al*, 1997). They include orchialgia (testicular pain), penile pain, prostate pain and perineal pain. Wesselmann *et al* (1997) stated that some pain relief can be provided by a multidisciplinary approach using pain medications, local treatment regimens, physiotherapy and psychological interventions.

Orchialgia

Orchialgia is pain in one or both testicles. Hayden (1993) and Holland *et al* (1994) treated orchialgia with transcutaneous electrical nerve stimulation (TENS) and considered the treatment beneficial.

Penile pain

Penile pain may be caused by penile prothesis surgery, intracavernosal injections or circumcision, and may have a psychological aspect (Wesselmann *et al*, 1997). There have not been any psychological studies of penile pain which are independent of other urogenital pain disorders. Causative conditions are paraphimosis (constriction of the glans penis by a tight foreskin), Peyronie's disease (penile deformity caused by fibrous tissue plaques which develop in the cavernous tissues), priapism (prolonged, painful penile erection lasting more than 4 h) and herpes genitalis. Penile pain may be relieved if the underlying cause is treated (Gee *et al*, 1990).

Prostatitis

Prostatitis occurs as a result of inflammation of the glandular portion of the prostate (Gray, 1992) causing discomfort in the rectal and suprapubic areas. The semen may be yellow or blood-stained. There are four types of prostatitis: acute bacterial, chronic bacterial, non-bacterial (prostatosis) and non-bacterial prostatodynia. Acute and chronic bacterial prostatitis occur as a result of ascending bacteria via the urethra. The causal agents of non-bacterial prostatitis and prostatodynia have not been identified.

The symptoms of prostatitis may be malaise and fever in the acute stage before the onset of dysuria, urgency, frequency and obstructive voiding. In both the acute and chronic stages, there may be pelvic pain.

Treatment for both bacterial and non-bacterial prostatitis is modestly effective. Antibiotics are used for bacterial prostatitis. Non-bacterial prostatitis has been treated in a clinical study of eight men with pulsed short-wave therapy (Singh *et al*, 1997). They used a drum electrode to the prostate gland. Each patient received eight treatments of 20 min duration and received treatment twice a week. Most of the men benefited from the treatment with four men showing complete relief of their symptoms. Only one man received no benefit. Chronic LUTS in young men are often misdiagnosed as non-bacterial prostatitis. Kaplan *et al* (1997) performed urodynamic studies on 43 men 23–50 years old with misdiagnosed chronic prostatitis and found contraction of the external urinary sphincter during voiding (pseudodyssynergia) to be the cause of functional bladder outlet obstruction. Six months of behaviour modification and biofeedback was successful in decreasing symptoms in 35 of these patients (83%). Without a control group it is impossible to say how many men would have improved naturally during that time.

Prostatodynia

Prostatodynia is non-bacterial inflammation of the prostate and urethra. Segura *et al* (1979) used pelvic floor relaxation techniques and rectal diathermy for patients with prostatodynia. Singh *et al* (1997) used short-wave therapy for this condition but studied only a small sample of men.

Perineal pain

Perineal pain may be present in patients with orchialgia and prostatody-nia (Wesselmann *et al*, 1997). Bensignor *et al* (1996) suggested that perineal pain was caused by pudendal nerve entrapment and Robert *et al* (1993) stated that surgical neurolysis-transposition of the pudendal nerve may have resulted in pain reduction.

Pain from cancer

It is important to note that there are no symptoms with prostate and blad-der cancer in the early stages. The first sign of bladder cancer is haema-turia. No two cancers are the same. In the later stages of prostate cancer there are symptoms of hip, leg and back pain which may be mistaken for arthritis.

Proctalgia fugax

Proctalgia fugax causes rectal pain due to spasm of the anal sphincter. This can sometimes be alleviated by sitting on the toilet and bearing down as if voiding faeces, thereby relaxing the anal sphincter.

Summary

Pelvic pain includes orchialgia (testicular pain), penile pain, prostatody-nia and perineal pain. Pain may be relieved if the underlying cause is treated. Some pain relief can be provided using pain medications, local treatment regimens, physiotherapy and psychological interventions.

CHAPTER 7

Patient assessment

Key points

- A detailed subjective and objective assessment is necessary in order to make a diagnosis.
- Urinalysis, uroflow and post-void residual examination contribute to a clear diagnosis.
- A digital rectal assessment will reveal the strength and endurance of the PFMs.

Subjective assessment

Before a diagnosis can be made, and before treatment can be commenced, a subjective and objective assessment is required (Dorey, 2000f). The subjective assessment is based on the patient's account of his symptoms. The Male Subjective Continence Assessment Form is shown in Appendix 1. The subjective assessment should include questions in the following categories.

Patient details

Patient details should include the patient's age, occupation, hobbies and activities in order to make a lifestyle evaluation.

Main problem

It is necessary to have knowledge of the severity and duration of the main problem, the limitation of activities, quality of life (QOL) and bothersome rating (0–10) caused by the main problem.

Symptoms

Questions should then be asked in order to evaluate the presenting symptoms of stress incontinence, frequency, nocturia, urgency, urge incontinence plus the factors provoking leakage (provoking factors), and nocturnal enuresis. In order to have knowledge of voiding (obstructive) symptoms, questions should be asked concerning: the flow rate, any difficulty starting voiding, any difficulty maintaining the stream, the strength of the stream, voided volumes (large or small), the presence of terminal dribble and whether the bladder feels empty after micturition. Do patients perform a Credé maneouvre (leaning forwards and pressing on the lower abdomen while straining to void urine)? Patients should be asked if they feel a sensation to void again on moving as this may indicate double void instability (when a detrusor contraction causes leakage after micturition). It is helpful to know if the patient has a sensation of voiding and an awareness of leaking. Does the patient have post-micturition dribble (PMD) or constant dribble? Is it painful to pass urine and is the urine dark, smelly, smoky, or containing blood? Any indication of pain in the pelvic area may be marked on a body chart.

Duration and severity of symptoms

The duration of each symptom needs to be noted plus the improvement or deterioration to date. The severity of each symptom can be marked on a visual analogue scale, from 0 (no problem) to 10 (severe problem).

Amount of leakage

The amount of leakage may be ascertained from a description by the patient and may be described as a few drops, or a medium or large leakage, the number of pads used per day, their size and whether the pads are damp, wet or soaked. Does the patient have an appliance and leg bag, use intermittent catheterisation or have an in-dwelling catheter?

Frequency of leakage

What is the frequency of leakage: is it daily, once a week or once a month? When does the leakage occur? Is the leakage provoked by coughing, sneezing, shouting, walking, moving, running water, caffeine, alcohol, medications or some other trigger?

Urine stop test

Can the patient stop or slow down the flow of urine mid-stream? This question provides the opportunity to explain that this exercise can lead to retention of urine, counteracts the normal micturition reflexes and therefore should not be practised.

Bowel activity

Does the patient suffer from constipation, strain to defaecate or practise digital evacuation? How many times a week does defaecation occur? Are the faeces liquid, soft or firm? Is there faecal urgency, faecal incontinence or incontinence of flatus? Does the patient use laxatives and does he have a balanced diet with sufficient fluids?

Surgical history

It is necessary to know the dates and outcomes of transuretheral resection of the prostate (TURP) and any repeat TURPs, radical prostatectomy, the presence of a urethral stricture and any other abdominal or relevant surgery.

Medical history

It is of interest to know if there are any family history trends. Has the patient suffered from prostatitis: how often, and was it acute or chronic? Has he had acute or chronic cystitis and with how many episodes? Is he allergic to latex, running the risk of anaphylactic shock if the therapist uses latex gloves? There is a high incidence of latex allergy among patients who have undergone multiple surgery for urinary bladder exstrophy (see Exstrophy of bladder, Chapter 2), and a significant correlation between latex sensitisation and the number and duration of surgical procedures and intermittent catheterisation (De Castro *et al*, 1999). Does he have any metal implants? Electrical stimulation is contra-indicated if there is metal in the field, which may concentrate the current and produce a burn. Does he smoke, have respiratory problems, or cough which exacerbates incontinence? Does he take anticholinergic medication (tolterodine or oxybutynin), alpha blockers such as doxazosin mesylate (Cardura), 5-alpha inhibitors? Is he on anti-androgen treatment or any other medication? What are the effect and side-effects of the medication? Has he undergone or is he undergoing radiotherapy? Is there a neurological problem such as diabetes, multiple sclerosis or Parkinson's disease, or a severe cervical or lumbar spine problem with a neurological deficit?

Previous treatment

Has the patient had previous conservative treatment and what was the outcome?

Body mass index

What is the patient's height and weight and what is his body mass index (BMI)?

BMI = weight (kg)/[height (m)]^2
BMI >25: overweight
BMI >30: seriously overweight
BMI >41: dangerously overweight

Sexual problems

Does the patient have difficulty achieving or maintaining penile erection? (see Chapters 10 and 11).

Functional factors

Is the patient able to stand for urination? Does he have adequate mobility and dexterity? Are there any environmental problems which make access to the toilet difficult? Is he cognitively impaired or having psychological problems and is there a patient support network of carers?

Motivation

Does the patient have the ability and motivation to incorporate the therapy into his lifestyle in order to comply with an exercise programme or with lifestyle changes?

Medical investigations

A full assessment also includes a urinalysis of mid-stream urine to eliminate urinary infection; a uroflow to monitor the force of the stream during micturition; and a post-void residual examination using bladder ultrasound to ensure bladder emptying. Other tests of interest are: PSA, urodynamics to diagnose genuine stress incontinence, urge incontinence and a low compliance bladder; and flexible cystoscopy for the diagnosis of strictures and bladder tumours. A 24 h pad test is useful before treatment and then at discharge as an outcome measure.

Frequency/volume chart

A frequency/volume (F/V) chart can provide detailed information of: the frequency of voiding, the maximum voided volume, the minimum voided volume, the amount of fluid intake, the amount of caffeine and alcohol intake, the amount of urinary output, the time of going to bed, the amount voided at night, the frequency of leakage and the number of pads used a day. It aids the diagnosis between urge incontinence, usually with attendant frequency and nocturia, and stress incontinence (see Tables 7.1 and 7.2).

Table 7.1 Frequency/volume chart of a man with stress incontinence

Frequency/volume chart

Name _____   Date _____

Time	Tick voiding urine	Amount voided (ml)	Tick leak	Type of drink	Amount drunk (ml)	Pad change	Comments: 'almost dry' 'damp' 'wet' or 'soaked'
6 am	√	470	√	Tea	250		Walked to bathroom –Wet
7 am							
8 am	√						
9 am							
10 am	√	260		Coffee	250		
11 am							
12 pm							
1 pm	√	250		Soup	150		
2 pm							
3 pm			√			√	Lifted rubbish - Wet
4 pm	√	200		Tea	200		
5 pm							
6 pm	√	200					
7 pm				Wine	250		
8 pm				Coffee	200		
9 pm							
10 pm			√	Water	200	√	Coughed – Damp
11 pm	√	350					
12 am							
1 am							
2 am							
3 am							
4 am							
5 am							
Totals	7	1730	3		1500	2	

Please bring your completed 3-day diary with you to your next appointment

There is some controversy concerning the number of days a F/V chart should be completed. Abrams *et al* (1997) advocated completion of the chart for 7 days and nights. It should include days at work, though this may lead to lack of patient compliance. It could be argued that an accurate 2–3 day F/V chart could pose less inconvenience to the patient and thereby gain patient compliance. It could be repeated at intervals to show progress.

Table 7.2 Frequency/volume chart of a man with urge incontinence

Frequency/volume chart

Name _____   Date _____

Time	Tick voiding urine	Amount voided (ml)	Tick leak	Type of drink	Amount drunk (ml)	Pad change	Comments: 'almost dry' 'damp' 'wet' or 'soaked'
6 am	√	130	√	Tea	250		Rushed to bath room
7 am	√	150					
8 am	√	50		Tea	250		
9 am	√	80					
10 am	√√	100	√	Coffee	250	√	Urgency – wet
11 am	√√	90	√			√	Urgency – damp
12 pm	√	120		Orange	200		
1 pm	√	140					
2 pm	√	60					
3 pm	√	150		Tea	200		
4 pm	√	100	√				Damp
5 pm	√	80					
6 pm							
7 pm	√	150	√	Beer	500	√	Urgency – soaked
8 pm							
9 pm							
10 pm	√	120		Water	100		
11 pm							
12 am							
1 am							
2 am							
3 am							
4 am							
5 am							
Totals	16	1520	5		1750	3	

Please bring your completed 3-day diary with you to your next appointment

Bladder diary

A bladder diary is a term used when the patient keeps a record of just the urine ouput and not the fluid intake. It fails to provide information on the amount, type and timing of fluid intake.

Objective assessment

The patient is given the opportunity to visit the toilet before the objective assessment. The objective assessment is an assessment of the patient's condition based on what the therapist observes (Dorey, 2000a). The Male Objective Continence Assessment Form is in Appendix 1.

The patient should be given the opportunity to be chaperoned by a partner, a friend or a member of staff. The objective assessment should always begin with an explanation of the reasons into the need for a digital rectal examination (DRE). It should be explained that it is necessary to know whether the muscles which can control continence are working equally on the right side and the left side of the pelvic floor. The strength and endurance of these muscles can best be assessed by palpating them, the method of exercising can be checked and the correct amount of exercise given. The skin sensation and integrity can also be checked. If the patient declines a DRE, he may allow a perineal examination but he should not be persuaded against his wishes. Following this detailed explanation, the patient must give informed consent to the objective examination and the consent must be entered in the patient notes. At this stage he should be given the opportunity to visit the toilet. For the objective examination, the patient should be lying on his back with two pillows under his head, his knees bent and his feet on the plinth without his underwear but with a sheet, towel or paper sheet over his pelvis. He may retain his sheath and drainage system if he has one.

Abdominal examination

In the supine lying position the abdomen is palpated for pain, pelvic masses, and bladder distension. Abdominal examination requires training and practice under medical supervision. Any abnormalities require referral to a GP or urologist.

The ultrasound bladder scan can be performed in this position.

Perineal examination

Observe the pelvic area in the crook lying position for congenital abnormalities such as hypospadias, epispadias, enlarged testis, warts, haemorrhoids or tumours. The skin condition should be examined for redness, infection and excoriation in the penile, perineal, scrotal and anal areas. All evidence should be recorded.

The patient may then be asked to tighten the anus as if to prevent wind escaping while the anal wink is observed. Then he can be asked to tighten at the front as if to prevent the flow of urine and feel a scrotal lift and the base of the penis lift towards the abdomen. After this, he is asked to give an unguarded cough which may provide evidence of leakage. He is then requested to cough while he is tightening his pelvic floor muscles (PFMs) to prevent leakage, which may provide evidence of urinary control.

The fourth sacral (S4) dermatome may be tested using a cotton wool bud or a gloved finger and gently stroking either side of the anus and either side of the perineum while asking the patient to describe what he feels. If there is neurological deficit, S2 dermatome may be checked on the lateral surface of the buttock, lateral thigh, posterior calf and plantar heel and S3 dermatome may be checked on the upper two-thirds of the inner surface of the thigh (see Figure 2.7). The knee jerk, ankle jerk and plantar reflexes should be tested if neurological impairment is suspected. If there is neurological impairment, the bulbocavernosus reflex may be tested during the DRE. The patient should be forewarned. Using gloves, the therapist uses the thumb and forefinger to exert gentle pressure on the glans penis during a DRE. If the bulbocavernosus reflex does not elicit an anal sphincter contraction, there is neurological impairment.

Digital rectal examination

The therapist approximates a gloved index finger covered amply with lubricating gel to the anal meatus, allowing the patient to feel the gel. The patient is then asked to bear down on to the finger as if he is letting wind escape. While the patient is bearing down, the finger is inserted straight, in a cephalad direction (towards the head) with the finger pad towards the coccyx. The finger can then be introduced to 1–2 cm from the meatus in order to assess the integrity and tone of the external anal sphincter (Dixon et al, 1997). Any areas of pain should be noted. With a lax sphincter, it may be possible to feel areas of scar tissue in the external anal sphincter where there is no muscle contraction. The patient should be asked to contract the anus and hold for 5 s, while the therapist grades the strength of the contraction and notes the duration of the hold in seconds. This can be repeated up to five times and then the ability to perform fast contractions noted. The examining finger can then be introduced to

3–4 cm from the meatus and the anterior pull of puborectalis gently felt at the anorectal angle. This muscle is then graded, as for any voluntary muscle in the body, 0–5 for muscle strength, for the duration of the hold and for the ability to perform fast contractions. From this DRE, the anal sphincter and the puborectalis can then be assessed and recorded using the modified Oxford scale (Laycock, 1994) (see Table 7.3).

Urodynamics

Urodynamic investigations study the bladder pressure during filling and voiding, its capacity and flow rate. Cystometric measurements are plotted on a graph or cystometrogram. Patients first sit on a commode over a uroflowmeter to measure the urinary flow rate (see Figure 4.1). After voiding, two catheters are introduced into the bladder; one to fill the bladder and one attached to a pressure sensor to monitor the bladder pressure. A third catheter with a pressure sensor is introduced into the rectum to measure the intra-abdominal pressure. The pressure of the detrusor muscle is calculated by subtracting the rectal pressure from the intravesical bladder pressure:

detrusor muscle pressure = bladder pressure – abdominal pressure.

The bladder is filled with saline or a similar filling medium at room temperature and the patient is asked to indicate his first desire to void. The man is asked to 'hold on' unless he feels undue discomfort. He may be asked to cough or stand up or walk on the spot in order to provoke evidence. A bladder contraction and leakage of urine demonstrates detrusor instability whereas leakage of urine on activity with no bladder contraction demonstrates genuine stress incontinence. He is asked to report when he experiences a strong desire to void and, when he cannot hold on, he is asked to void over the flowmeter once more.

Table 7.3 Assessment of strength of the pelvic floor muscles (Laycock, 1994 reproduced with permission)

Description	Grade
Nil	0
Flicker	1
Weak	2
Moderate	3
Good	4
Strong	5

A normal bladder will allow filling until the maximum capacity of 400–600 ml is reached (see Figure 7.1). The rise in detrusor pressure should be minimal as the normal bladder stretches to accommodate the filling medium.

Figure 7.2b shows a cystometrogram trace of a man with detrusor instability. Note the sharp increase in bladder pressure provoked by a cough.

Figure 7.2c shows a cystometrogram trace of a man with stress incontinence. Note the detrusor pressure does not rise with coughing.

Videourodynamics with contrast medium allows visualisation of the bladder, bladder neck and urethra. Ambulatory urodynamics is also utilised in some centres.

Chaudry *et al* (1997) states that many men with apparent lower urinary tract obstruction would have had inappropriate treatment if their management relied solely on symptom scoring, flow rate and residual

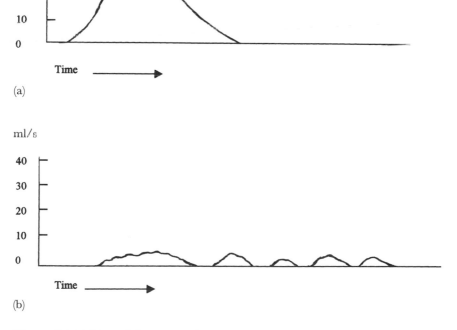

Figure 7.1 (a) Normal flow curve. (b) Reduced flow due to obstruction or poor bladder contraction.

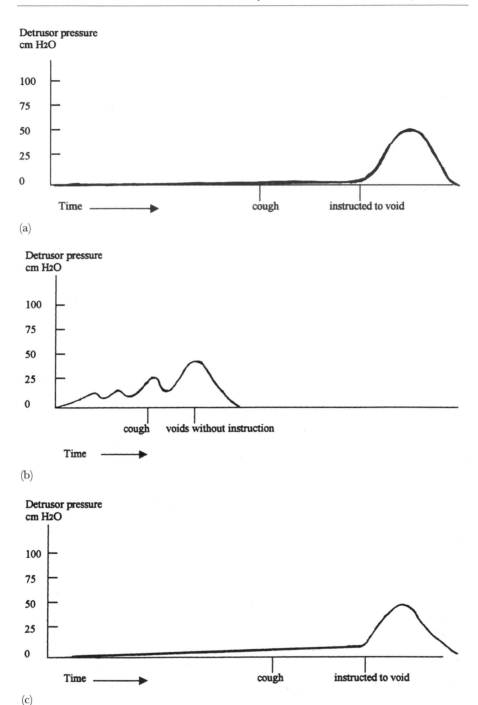

Figure 7.2 Cystometrogram traces: (a) Normal. (b) Detrusor instability. (c) Stress incontinence.

urine measurement. They stated that urodynamics should be used in order to provide a predictable subjective and objective outcome of treatment after a prostatectomy. Urodynamic findings may not be comparable with history taking. Vereecken and Wouters (1988) found that there was discrepancy in about a third of cases. They considered that this may be due either to poor history taking or to the artificial conditions of the examination. Ambulatory urodynamics may provide a better understanding of bladder dysfunction but there were still pitfalls in the presence of artefacts (irregular readings) and the incidence of catheter expulsion during micturition.

Summary

A detailed subjective and objective assessment is necessary in order to make a diagnosis. A digital rectal assessment will reveal the strength, endurance and ability to perform fast contractions of the pelvic floor muscles. A frequency/volume chart provides valuable information.

Urodynamic investigations study the bladder pressure during filling and voiding, its capacity and flow rate.

CHAPTER 8

Conservative treatment

Key points

- Frequency, nocturia, urgency, urge incontinence, stress incontinence, PMD and post-prostatectomy incontinence can be treated conservatively.
- Treatment regimes have been compiled from the data produced from a Delphi study using 14 experts from 5 countries.
- Treatment progression is patient specific and dependent on ongoing assessment.

Conservative treatment for men with lower urinary tract symptoms

Pelvic floor muscle exercises (PFMEs), biofeedback, bladder training, electrical stimulation, behavioural strategies and advice have all been utilised for the treatment of men with lower urinary tract symptoms (LUTS) (Dorey, 1999, 2000b). Moore and Dorey (1999) in a literature review found the benefits in men were not well researched although in non-randomised and non-controlled trials, the results appeared encouraging (Sotiropoulus *et al*, 1976; Krauss and Lilien, 1981; Burgio *et al*, 1989; Meaglia *et al*, 1990; Jackson *et al*, 1996; Mathewson-Chapman, 1997; Chang *et al*, 1998) (see Table 8.1).

Two of the three recent randomised, controlled trials (RCTs) supported the intervention of physiotherapy treatment for men with post-micturition dribble (PMD) (Paterson *et al*, 1997) and post-prostatectomy urinary incontinence (Van Kampen *et al*, 2000).

Table 8.1 Conservative physiotherapy treatment for urinary incontinence in men (Moore and Dorey, 1999)

Classification	Symptoms	Treatment options
Urge incontinence (overactive bladder)	Involuntary loss of urine associated with a strong desire to void; may be due to detrusor instability	Bladder training Lifestyle adjustments Pelvic floor muscle exercises Biofeedback Electrical stimulation (Anticholinergic medications)
Stress incontinence	Involuntary loss of urine on physical exertion or increase in intra-abdominal pressure due to sphincter deficiency	Pelvic floor muscle exercises The 'Knack' Bulbar urethral massage Biofeedback Electrical stimulation
Mixed incontinence (urge and stress)	Urge and stress symptoms	Combination of the above
Post-micturition dribble	Loss of urine post micturition due to urine retention in the bulbar part of the urethra	Pelvic floor muscle exercises 'Squeeze out' contraction Bulbar urethral massage
Post-prostatectomy incontinence	Symptoms of urge or stress incontinence or PMD	Pre-operative PFMEs Treat as stress or urge incontinence according to the symptoms Post-operative scar tissue massage
Overflow	Involuntary loss of urine associated with over-distension of the bladder due to acontractile or underactive detrusor or bladder outlet obstruction	Intermittent self-catheterisation (relief of obstruction)
Functional incontinence	Due to functional problems exacerbating existing bladder problems, e.g. poor mobility, difficult clothing, confusion	Improve environment Social care Lifestyle adaptations Clothing adaptations Continence aids

Patient education

Most men know little about the prostate gland or its anatomical location. Many lack knowledge of any potential medical problems or the treatments available (Smith, 1997). In a controlled clinical trial of urinary incontinence, a telephone interview involving 1140 participants aged 65 years and older in Massachusetts, USA, Branch *et al* (1994) found that there were substantial gaps in older people's knowledge of urinary incontinence, especially among men aged 85 years and older and those with lower education levels.

All members of the healthcare team have a responsibility to impart health education in the form of verbal instruction, booklets, diagrams and videos, to help people make informed decisions about their lifestyle and health (Edmonds, 1991). In a study by the Royal Commission of the NHS (1978), 95% of 500 patients questioned found that written information was beneficial and helped to relieve anxiety. Reading matter should have simple terminology and large print.

All treatment should commence with an explanation of the patient's condition and the treatment options available. It is helpful to use a model of the male pelvis complete with musculature in order to explain the anatomy and physiology.

Stress incontinence

Stress incontinence in men may occur as a result of sphincter damage following a prostatectomy (Donnellan *et al*, 1997). The internal sphincter is damaged in all forms of prostatectomy. Physiotherapy has the potential to be effective in alleviating the stress incontinence caused by an incompetent urethral sphincter by the use of PFMEs similar to those used in the treatment of women (Bø, 1995).

Pelvic floor muscle exercises

The passive urethral mucosal seal is actively compressed by the external urethral sphincter and PFMs (Harrison and Abrams, 1994). PFMEs are non-invasive and are not associated with serious complications and may be appropriate for patients with stress incontinence who wish to avoid surgery (Gray, 1992). These exercises should be individually taught to make sure the patient is lifting up the pelvic floor and not bearing down as if defaecating (i.e. performing a valsalva manoeuvre). The amount and progression of patient-specific pelvic floor exercise is determined by individual assessment and digital rectal examination (DRE). Men can be encouraged to tighten and lift the PFMs as in the control of flatus or the prevention of urine flow, and can practise in front of a mirror to observe a visible dip in the angle at the base of the penis and a scrotal lift (Paterson *et al*, 1997; Moore *et al*, 1999). Patients can be taught to palpate a contraction of the ischiocavernosus muscle at the perineum 2 cm medially and 2 cm anteriorly to the ischial tuberosity (see Figure 8.1).

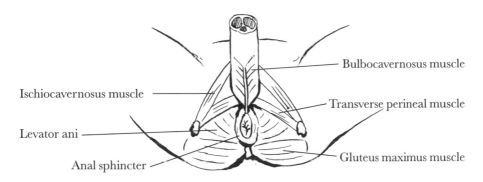

Figure 8.1 Male superficial pelvic floor muscles.

The convenient positions for practising PFMEs are in crook lying with knees bent and the knees apart; standing with feet apart; and sitting with knees apart (Burgio *et al*, 1989; Paterson *et al*, 1997; Van Kampen *et al*, 2000; Moore *et al*, 1999). It is the intensity rather than frequency of work that is important, as maximal voluntary effort causes muscle hypertrophy and increased muscle strength (Guyton, 1986; Dinubile, 1991; Bø, 1994). In order to achieve full fitness, PFMEs should be taught for endurance as well as for muscle strength by submaximal contractions (Guyton, 1986). Muscle training, therefore, depends on the motivation of the patient and his adherence to the pelvic floor muscle exercise regimen (Jackson *et al*, 1996). It may help patients to keep an exercise diary.

Pelvic floor muscle strength

Muscle strength development is achieved by the combination of the recruitment of a greater number of motor units, a higher frequency of excitation and muscle hypertrophy. With increasing load, the recruitment of additional and increasingly larger motor units takes place. When additional force is demanded, both slow- and fast-twitch fibres are recruited. The intensity rather than the frequency of work is important and high tension must be created to increase strength. Guyton (1986) stated that muscle strength was increased by maximal voluntary effort which caused muscle hypertrophy. A contraction as close to maximum as possible is required to create high tension in order to address the principles of overload and specificity (DiNubile, 1991; Bø, 1994). There is controversy over the outcomes of increased muscle strength. In one trial (Jackson *et al*, 1996) pelvic floor muscle strength did not predict the outcome following radical prostatectomy. This may have been because the outcome was measured by digital assessment. Haslam *et al* (1998) found that inter-tester reliability could not be assured unless appropriate training was provided. Jackson *et al* (1996) used a scale which graded from 0 (no palpable contraction) to 3 (strong) and did not give the range of muscle strength grades that the more generally used scale of 0–5 would have done (see Table 7.3).

As with any voluntary muscle training, a weak muscle is strengthened to perform the required task. This means attaining and then maintaining a level of fitness. McArdle *et al* (1991) defined fitness as a set of attributes that relate to the ability to perform physical activity. The components of fitness are shown in Table 8.2 (Norris, 1997).

Pelvic floor muscle endurance

In order to achieve full fitness, PFMEs should be taught for endurance as well as for muscle strength. Guyton (1986) stated that endurance is the time limit of a person's ability to maintain either a static (isometric) force or a power level of dynamic exercise. He also found that endurance was improved by submaximal repetitive contractions. Both static and dynamic endurance are necessary for normal pelvic floor performance. Static endurance is defined as the interval in which a maximal or submaximal contraction can be maintained whereas dynamic endurance is the number of contractions performed with constant frequency and load before exhaustion occurs (Christensen and Hulgang-Frederiksen, 1998).

'The knack'

'The knack' is the ability to initiate a PFM contraction sufficiently far in advance of an intra-abdominal pressure rise (Ashton-Miller and DeLancey, 1996). It is called 'the knack' in recognition of the motor control skill required. There is controversy about the voluntary control

Table 8.2 Components of fitness (S factors) (Norris, 1997)

Stamina
Suppleness
Strength
Speed
Skill
Specificity

and innervation of the urinary sphincter. It may be that it contracts with the PFMs, but this action has not been identified. The key to bladder control may be in the urethral sphincter 'guarding reflex' identified in cats (Garry et al, 1959). Park et al (1997) revisited the guarding reflex and stated that pelvic floor exercises may affect continence by increasing the ability to 'guard' or contract quickly during times of increased intra-abdominal pressure. Gordon and Logue (1985) found that the upright position when standing and walking stimulated the pelvic floor reflex, and Mahony et al (1977) stated that increased pelvic floor tone should diminish nocturia.

Specific home exercise programme

No research has been conducted that gives clear indications of the number of PFMEs to perform in order to build up muscle bulk, strength and endurance. Kegel (1956) instructed female patients to exercise the PFMs 2–3 times a day for 20 min using a perineometer. In addition, patients performed PFMEs 5–10 times every half hour during the day. This amounted to about 300 contractions a day. In muscle building, it is the quality not the quantity that is important. Some physiotherapists recommend maximal home exercises twice a day in crook lying, sitting and standing, and report considerable improvement. Randomised controlled trials are needed to ascertain the number of repetitions needed to gain optimum relief of the symptoms. When men are given PFMEs to perform every hour, they will feel guilty if they are unable to comply. Many therapists give patients more exercises than they need in the hope of getting a degree of compliance. In order to gain compliance, it is surely better to have an honest agreement with the patient and let him know the exact number of contractions required.

Motivation and compliance

Muscle training depends on the motivation of the patient and the adherence to the pelvic floor exercise regimen (Jackson et al, 1996). Knight and Laycock (1994) stated that the success of PFMEs in women depended on a high level of patient motivation and compliance. Wilson et al (1987) concluded that female patients performed PFMEs better when they attended outpatient departments and were less motivated when left to a scheme of home exercises. However, Holley et al (1995) found that only 1 out of 10 women suffering from genuine stress incontinence were sufficiently motivated to perform PFME after 5 years.

Pelvic floor muscle exercises for stress incontinence

PFMEs should be patient specific. The hold time in seconds is ascertained from the digital rectal assessment. The rest time should exceed the hold time to allow muscle fibre recovery. There is no evidence for an optimum number of repeat contractions, but the objective assessment will help determine what is appropriate for each patient. The quality of contraction is more important than the quantity. Exercises should be practised every day and include some fast and some slow contractions. A typical programme practised twice a day could be: three maximum contractions in crook lying, three maximum contractions in sitting and three maximum contractions in standing, held for the length of time in seconds specific to the patient. However, this is only a guide. Some contractions may be activated quickly and some slowly. The patient can also be encouraged to lift the pelvic floor up 50% of their maximum while walking, to encourage postural support. Men can be taught 'the knack' of tightening the PFMs before activities which increase the intra-abdominal pressure such as coughing, sneezing, rising from sitting or lifting (Ashton-Miller and DeLancey, 1996).

Biofeedback treatment for stress incontinence

Biofeedback is a mechanism by which the patient is more aware of pelvic floor muscle activity and encourages greater muscular effort (Burgio *et al*, 1989; Knight and Laycock, 1994; Jackson *et al*, 1996; Van Kampen *et al*, 1998). Many patients are unable to contract their pelvic floor or do not understand the maximal effort needed. Biofeedback can often provide the necessary awareness for muscle re-education. There are three recognised methods of biofeedback: digital, manometric (pressure) and electromyographic (Bump *et al*, 1991; Haslam, 1999). The three biofeedback methods have been studied and compared and they appear to correlate well with one another (Haslam, 1999).

Digital rectal biofeedback

A lubricated gloved index finger can be used during a digital rectal examination to monitor the strength and endurance of the external anal sphincter and the puborectalis muscle (see Chapter 7, Patient assessment). The information can then be communicated to the patient in order to provide feedback and encouragement.

Manometric biofeedback

A rectal pressure probe can be used to monitor muscle activity and provide manometric (pressure) biofeedback. The rectal probe may be attached to a perincometer with a visual display (see Figure 8.2). Sophisticated computerised equipment with a coloured visual display screen, audible feedback, a variety of work and rest programmes, and printer is considered the gold standard by many therapists (see Figure 8.3). This equipment may also be used for electromyography (EMG) and electrical stimulation. The patient should be placed in crook lying with his knees bent and apart with a sheet or paper sheet over his pelvis. He should be able to see and hear the monitor screen. The probe should be covered

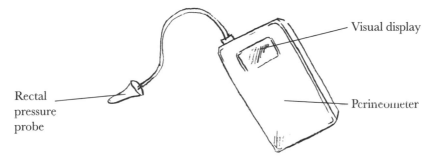

Figure 8.2 Perineometer with rectal pressure probe.

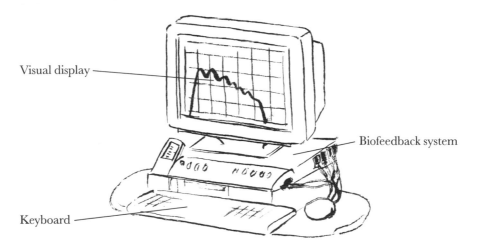

Figure 8.3 Computerised biofeedback equipment.

with a condom, lubricated with gel and approximated to the patient's anus. The patient is then asked to bear down as if releasing flatus while the probe is gently inserted. The probe needs to be held in a position which records maximal readings and prevents it from slipping out (see Figure 8.4). The difficulty with a rectal pressure probe is that it records the activity of both the anal sphincter and the puborectalis muscle. It is important to record the activity of the puborectalis muscle which lies above and is integrated with the pubococcygeus muscle which surrounds the external urethral sphincter.

The pressure is usually measured in bars or numerical units on a perineometer or by centimetres of water (cm H_2O) or millimetres of mercury (mm Hg) on more accurate manometric equipment.

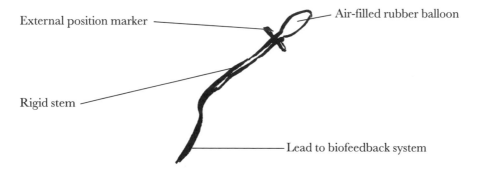

External position marker

Air-filled rubber balloon

Rigid stem

Lead to biofeedback system

Figure 8.4 Rectal probe for manometric (pressure) biofeedback.

Electromyographic biofeedback

EMG is the study of minute electrical potentials produced by depolarisation of the muscle membrane (Siroky, 1996). Bioelectric activity of the muscles can be recorded using either a needle sensor, a rectal probe or surface sensors. The bioelectric activity is measured in units of microvolts (μV).

- **Needle EMG**, which is invasive and may be painful, is currently out of the scope of nurses and physiotherapists.
- The **rectal probe** (which may also be used for electrical stimulation) is easier to apply using lubricating gel, but most probes need to be held by the therapist to prevent slippage. New shaped rectal electrodes fit snugly into position and allow ambulatory use (Figure 8.5). Rectal probes are strictly for single patient use. The rectal probes are attached to a computerised biofeedback machine, which will monitor

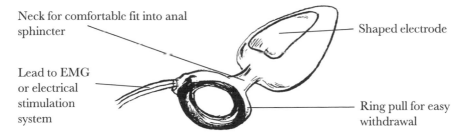

Neck for comfortable fit into anal sphincter

Lead to EMG or electrical stimulation system

Shaped electrode

Ring pull for easy withdrawal

Figure 8.5 Rectal probe for EMG or electrical stimulation.

the bioelectric activity of the muscles by EMG biofeedback and provide a coloured visual display and sometimes an audible signal to encourage greater effort.

- **Surface sensors** may be used on the perineum. They can be used to monitor the activity of the pubococcygeus and the ischiococcygeus muscles. The skin needs to be cleansed with an alcohol swab to remove any oils that may prevent a good contact. It may be necessary to shave the area. Better contact is also made by using new surface sensors for each treatment. Two small sticky surface sensors may be placed longitudinally over the pubococcygeus and the ischiococcygeus muscle to be monitored by EMG and may be placed 1 cm lateral to the midline (see Figure 8.6). A third sensor may be placed over a bony point such as the sacrum or coccyx to act as a reference (grounding) to cut out extraneous 'noise' from the electrical activity of other muscles in the area. However, some EMG equipment use a triangular arrangement for all three sensors with the two active sensors longitudinal to the muscle fibres. One of the benefits of EMG is its use in functional positions. Problems associated with the use of EMG may be due to the size of the sensor pad or probe which may pick up electrical activity from the surrounding muscles. However, surface EMG is non-invasive, painless and can also be used as an initiator of cerebral control, a tool of assessment, a motivator and a method of recording; it can be used to both encourage and challenge the patient (Haslam, 1998). Manometric (pressure) or EMG biofeedback (Figure 8.7) is a useful adjunct to pelvic floor muscle re-education to stimulate greater patient effort.

Electrical stimulation for stress incontinence

There are two basic types of electrical stimulation which have been used on PFMs: maximal electrical stimulation and low intensity electrical stimulation.

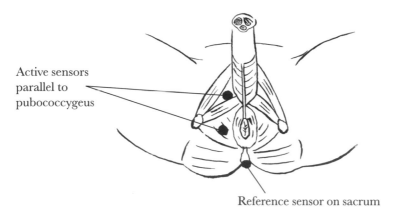

Active sensors
parallel to
pubococcygeus

Reference sensor on sacrum

Figure 8.6 Position of surface sensors for EMG biofeedback.

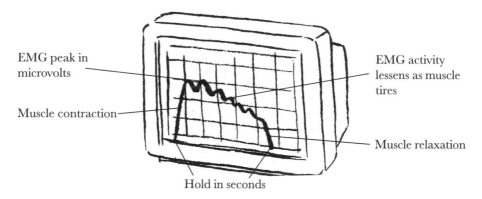

EMG peak in
microvolts

EMG activity
lessens as muscle
tires

Muscle contraction

Muscle relaxation

Hold in seconds

Figure 8.7 EMG biofeedback shown on a computer screen.

- **Maximal electrical stimulation** is applied pulsed at the maximum intensity tolerable for short periods of 20 min at a frequency of about 30 Hz to produce a tetanic contraction, and is used for stress incontinence in women (Jones, 1995).
- **Low intensity electrical stimulation** may be applied pulsed or continuous for several hours a day for several months. However, continuous low intensity electrical stimulation can lead to a conversion of muscle fibre type from fast-twitch (type 2) to slow-twitch (type 1) (Salmons and Henriksonn, 1981). This may produce an undesired effect as the recruitment of fast-twitch fibres of the PFMs is necessary during rises in intra-abdominal pressure.

Electrical stimulation of the PFMs may be delivered by rectal or surface electrodes. The rectal electrode contains positive and negative bands and is used alone. It is strictly for single patient use. Surface electrodes may be placed on the coccyx and the perineum or on either side of the perineal body as shown in Figure 8.8. Care should be taken to avoid burning, which may occur with small electrodes. Skin sensation should be tested before treatment and the skin should be viewed after treatment. Contra-indications to electrical stimulation are listed in Table 8.3.

Table 8.3 Contra-indications to electrical stimulation

Lack of consent
Patient is anxious
Patient lacks understanding
Any broken skin in the area
Any metal in the field (will concentrate the current and lead to a burn)
Patient with severe cardiac problems and/or with a pacemaker
Cancer
Loss of sensation
Poor circulation
Epilepsy
Recent surgery
Recent or recurrent haemorrhages

A current of sufficient amplitude will excite nerve and muscle tissue in its field, causing a muscular contraction. Electrical stimulation has been used for patients who are initially unable to contract the PFMs. However, Berghmans *et al* (1998) noted that in five randomised controlled trials (RCTs) in women, electrical stimulation was found to be no more effective than PFMEs alone. In fact, Knight and Laycock (1998) found that pulsed low intensity electrical stimulation may have a detrimental influence on female patients with genuine stress incontinence. In men, even less research has been conducted.

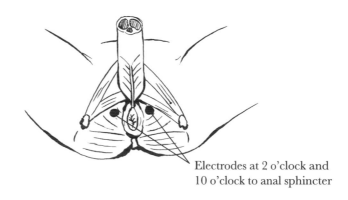

Electrodes at 2 o'clock and
10 o'clock to anal sphincter

Figure 8.8 Position of electrodes for electrical stimulation.

The real clinical benefit of electrical stimulation remains to be clarified. It may be that it can increase the circulation to the pelvic floor, or it may be useful to show patients how to initially contract the PFMs.

In women, electrical stimulation has been used for stress urinary incontinence at a frequency of 30–50 Hz. This wavelength produces a tetanic contraction with minimal risk of undue muscle fatigue, provided that the pulse train off-time is equal to or exceeds the on-time (Benton *et al*, 1981; Laycock *et al*, 1994). Knight and Laycock (1994) stated that a pulse width of 200 µs produced excitation at relatively low current intensity and was more comfortable than shorter pulse widths. They suggested that acute maximal electrical stimulation may benefit patients with very weak PFMs.

Electrical stimulation has been used for men with stress urinary incontinence after prostatectomy (Sotiropoulos *et al*, 1976; Krauss and Lilien, 1981; Hirakawa *et al*, 1993; Bennet *et al*, 1997; Moore, 1997). However, the treatment has been combined with PFMEs in two studies (Hirakawa *et al*, 1993; Moore *et al*, 1999) and the sample size in each case was small. In the only two RCTs, Bennett *et al* (1997) and Moore *et al* (1999) both found no improvement compared to control groups.

Urge incontinence

The filling symptoms of frequency, nocturia, urgency and urge incontinence can be treated with PFMEs, behavioural training and lifestyle changes, including advice on fluid intake (Burgio *et al*, 1989; Paterson *et al*, 1997; Dorey, 1998; Van Kampen *et al*, 1998).

Pelvic floor muscle exercises for urge incontinence

PFMEs can be used for urge incontinence to strengthen the pelvic floor musculature and regain the ability to control the urge to void urine. It is suggested that when the pelvic floor contracts the detrusor muscle will relax as a result of the activity of the perineopudendal facilitative reflex (Mahony *et al*, 1977) (see Chapter 3). Muscle training can be enhanced by the use of biofeedback, as discussed in the treatment for stress incontinence.

Electrical stimulation for urge incontinence

Urge incontinence may be treated with continuous maximal biphasic electrical stimulation at a frequency of 5–10 Hz with a pulse width of 200 µs for up to 20 min for urge suppression (Fall and Lindstrom, 1991;

Jones, 1994). Geirsson and Fall (1997) used stimulation parameters of 0.75 ms continuous biphasic waves with a frequency of 5 Hz in the treatment of detrusor instability in order to cause reflex inhibition of detrusor contractions. Some units provide intermittent biphasic electrical stimulation at 5–10 Hz which are used for urge incontinence.

Lifestyle changes and behavioural techniques for urge incontinence

There are several non-invasive techniques which individually or combined may improve the symptoms of frequency, nocturia, urgency and urge incontinence. These include bladder retraining, treating constipation, weight reduction, the adjustment of fluids, and the review of medications including diuretics. Techniques worked out in collaboration with other members of the healthcare team such as bowel management, weight loss, medication review and treatment of urinary tract infection may all improve symptoms. Education, attention to quantity, type and timing of fluid intake, avoiding constipation and delaying the urge to micturate are now considered part of lifestyle changes which can alter previous behaviour patterns. Because of the limitations of the latest research, current knowledge and practice is based on opinion and consensus but not on strong evidence.

Bladder training for urge incontinence

Bladder training (Frewen, 1979), also termed bladder retraining (Mahady and Begg, 1981), bladder drill (Elder and Stephenson, 1980), bladder re-education (Millard and Oldenburg, 1983) and urge suppression is a method of consciously suppressing the urge to void in order to delay micturition and increase functional bladder capacity (Wells, 1988). Frewen (1979) emphasised the psychological aspects of detrusor instability, which may be influenced by life events. Deferment techniques to delay voiding may be taught with strategies such as sitting on a hard surface, standing still, keeping calm, contracting the PFMs and distraction (see Table 8.4). Once the urge has abated, men will be able to

Table 8.4 Urge suppression techniques

Stand still or sit down on a hard surface
Relax the abdominal muscles
Keep calm
Contract the pelvic floor muscles
After the urge has disappeared continue previous activities

continue their activities, thus allowing their bladder to stretch and fill further. Patients undergoing bladder training need considerable encouragement, motivation and determination to succeed.

Fluid intake

Guyton (1986) stated that normal fluid intake averages 2300 ml per day, of which two-thirds (1518 ml) is direct fluid and the rest is a product of food digestion. Weisberg (1982) found a helpful gauge was 14–20 ml of fluid intake per pound of body weight. It may be more helpful to monitor the 24 h urine output, which should be about 1000–1500 ml. Normal intake should be increased during hot weather, with strenuous activity and when eating salty foods. No one should ever be thirsty. If the urine is dark, the patient should be encouraged to drink more fluid. However, some food products, vitamins and medication can affect the colour of urine. Beetroot makes urine pink, B vitamins make it yellow, and the urinary antiseptics gantrisin and pyridium make it red. Water is the best fluid to drink (see Table 9.1, page 93).

Moul (1998) listed foods and beverages which may irritate the bladder and may lead to overactivity. The foods include citrus products, tomato products, highly spiced foods, sugar, honey, chocolate and corn syrup, and the beverages include alcohol, colas, milk, coffee, tea and other drinks containing caffeine. Anecdotal reports suggest that caffeine reduction relieves symptoms in people with an overactive bladder. RCTs are needed to confirm the effect these products have on the bladder.

Diuretics

Natural diuretics are commonly xanthines, such as caffeine and theobromine, occurring primarily in beverages, which act chemically in the body to increase urine production. Caffeine occurs naturally in about 60 species of plants, most commonly coffee beans, tea leaves, cocoa seeds and the cola nut (Moore, 1990). Caffeine is also added to several over-the-counter medicines, to counteract the drowsiness that is a side-effect of the drug or to enhance analgesic absorption (Wells, 1988). Caffeine is a bladder irritant and stimulant with a diuretic effect. It also lowers urethral pressure (Palermo and Zimskind, 1977). It can cause the smooth muscle of the detrusor to contract with implications of nocturia, frequency, urgency and urge incontinence (Addison, 1997). Addison (1997) considered that men who are particularly at risk are those with detrusor instability or neurological disease, and the elderly. However, he stated that

caffeine should be reduced slowly in order to prevent withdrawal symptoms of headaches or drowsiness.

Cranberry juice

In the nineteeth century, the North American Indians used crushed cranberries as a herbal remedy for the treatment of urinary tract infections (Bodel *et al*, 1959; Moen, 1962). Although many studies have focused on the alteration in urinary pH (Fellers *et al*, 1933) or the increased hippuric acid levels (Bodel *et al*, 1959; Kinney and Blount, 1979), cranberry juice is also believed to have a bacteriostatic effect by affecting the adherence of certain organisms, in particular *Escherichia coli*, to the lining of the bladder (Beachy, 1981).

Avorn *et al* (1994) conducted an RCT with a sample of elderly women consuming either 300 ml of cranberry juice or a placebo. Results showed that cranberry juice reduced the occurrence of bacteriuria with pyuria.

Addison (1997) recommended cranberry juice for those patients with a high risk of urinary tract infection, those with cystitis from *E. coli*, patients with in-dwelling catheters, those undertaking intermittent self-catheterisation or those using sheath drainage. He considered that the recommendation of cranberry juice should be supported by written patient information and be monitored and recorded with dosage, patient instructions, contra-indications, side-effects and expected outcomes. There is controversy concerning the consumption of cranberry juice, as drinking in excess of 1 litre a day over a prolonged period may increase the risk of uric stone formation (Rogers, 1991). Other side-effects include gastritis, and for rheumatoid arthitis sufferers, increased joint pain, (Addison, 1997) and in patients with irritable bowel syndrome, diarrhoea (Leaver, 1996). Diabetics could find an increase in blood sugar level. For patients who simply do not like the taste, or find the juice too expensive, cranberry juice capsules can be purchased in health shops but there is no research on how they compare with the juice itself (Leaver, 1996).

Medication for urge incontinence

For men with severe urge incontinence or with nocturnal enuresis, anticholinergic medication may be helpful while they are receiving conservative treatment. Oxybutynin or tolterodine may be prescribed by the GP. Tolterodine (Detrusitol) has fewer side-effects than oxybutynin. The side-effects of both medications include a dry mouth, drowsiness, constipation and vision accommodation difficulties (see Chapter 9).

Acupuncture for urge incontinence

Acupuncture and electro-acupuncture have been used for urge incontinence. The treatment should be given by a physiotherapist or nurse who
is specialised in acupuncture. More research is needed in this area.

Post-prostatectomy incontinence

Post-prostatectomy incontinence should be treated according to the
presenting symptoms. Usually this is either stress incontinence or urge
incontinence but many patients may present with mixed incontinence
(both stress and urge incontinence).

Preoperative treatment

It would be useful for patients to receive PFME education before prostate
surgery. They could then increase the strength and endurance of the
PFMs and prevent or reduce incontinence after surgery. Patients benefit
by being taught pelvic floor exercises preoperatively when they are fit and
able to cope with learning a new skill. Unfortunately it is not always possible to provide a preoperative programme of strengthening exercises for
the PFMs as many patients do not present for treatment at this stage.
However, Sueppel (1998) realised the value of preoperative PFMEs and
taught patients prior to radical prostatectomy with encouraging results.
Bales et al (2000) found that biofeedback did not improve the outcome of
PFMEs on the return of urinary control in men undergoing radical
prosatectomy. However, both the treatment group and the control group
practised PFMEs four times a day and the treatment group only received
one biofeedback treatment. It is not clear from present research whether
preoperative PFMEs improve continence achievement. There is likely to
be a positive benefit from the relationship established between the therapist and the patient.

Postoperative treatment

After TURP or radical prostatectomy patients can gently tighten up the
PFMs immediately after surgery while they have an in-dwelling catheter,
provided the surgeon is in agreement. When the catheter has been
removed, a specific PFME programme should be practised. Following
surgery, patients may have iatrogenic stress incontinence due to sphincter
damage during surgery, or urge incontinence, or a combination of both
types. The 'knack' of tightening at times of increased intra-abdominal

pressure should be taught to cope with activities such as moving from sitting to standing, coughing and sneezing (Ashton-Miller and DeLancey, 1996).

In an RCT, 30 men undergoing TURP were taught PFMEs during an initial visit before surgery and encouraged to practise at home after surgery (Porru *et al*, 2001). Incontinence episodes and post-micturition dribbling (PMD) were significantly lower in the treatment group than in the controls at 1, 2, and 3 weeks ($p < 0.01$).

Post-micturition dribbling

Patients suffering from PMD can be taught a self-help technique called bulbar urethral massage or urethral milking to ease this distressing condition. After urinating, the patient places his fingers behind the scrotum and gently massages the bulbar urethra in a forwards and upwards direction in order to 'milk' the remaining urine from the urethra. It is helpful to use a diagram (see Figure 8.9) or an educational model. Tightening the PFMs prior to bulbar massage may help to prevent further leakage. In a randomised single-blind trial to test the efficacy of urethral milking, Paterson *et al* (1997) found PFMEs twice as effective as urethral milking and recommended pelvic floor exercises as a treatment for this condition. Contracting the PFMs after voiding may facilitate a contraction of the bulbocavernosus muscle, thus eliminating urine from the bulbar portion of the urethra.

Overflow incontinence

Clean intermittent self-catheterisation is used for patients with incomplete emptying due to an acontractile bladder, a hypotonic bladder or

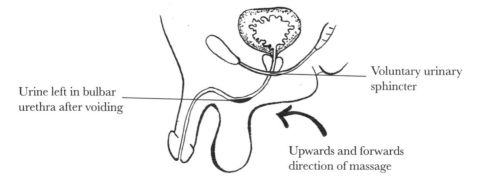

Voluntary urinary sphincter

Urine left in bulbar urethra after voiding

Upwards and forwards direction of massage

Figure 8.9 Bulbar massage for post-micturition dribble.

detrusor/sphincter dyssynergia. An acontractile bladder occurs when the smooth detrusor muscle fails to contract as a result of either lack of neurological control or overstretching. Overstretching may also cause pelvic nerve compression. The contraction from a hypotonic bladder may not be strong enough to completely empty the bladder. Detrusor/sphincter dyssynergia is due to neurological impairment and occurs when the detrusor muscle and sphincter contract simultaneously during voiding. This can result in retention of urine in the bladder.

Reflex incontinence

Reflex incontinence is usually the result of a neurological condition (e.g. spinal cord injury). The bladder fills and empties automatically by hyperreflexia, which is an uncontrolled reflex contraction. The treatment for reflex incontinence consists of clean intermittent self-catheterisation, a sheath drainage system or – as a last resort – an in-dwelling catheter. For patients who are permanently catheterised, a suprapubic catheter is more acceptable. Medication, in the form of anticholinergic drugs, or surgery, such as a clam ileocystoplasty, sphincterotomy for detrusor dyssynergia or sacral root stimulation by neuromodulation may be necessary.

- **Clam ileocystoplasty** is an operation in which a portion of the ileum is used to augment the bladder. This operation is designed to overcome detrusor hyperreflexia. The bladder is opened up like a clam and the portion of ileum with its own blood supply is sewn to the bladder to increase bladder capacity. However, the transplanted ileum continues to produce mucus, which may form a plug in the urethra causing retention. Some patients have problems emptying the bladder completely and need to use intermittent self-catheterisation.
- **Sacral nerve modulation** is performed by surgically implanting an electrode into the third sacral foramina to stimulate the third sacral nerve (S3) in order to maintain continence (Tanagho, 1990). The electrode is connected to an implantable pulse generator (stimulator) implanted into the abdominal cavity. The device may be turned on to allow bladder filling and off to allow voiding with a magnet held over the stimulator. Problems of infection, migration of the electrodes and pain can occur after surgery.

Extra-urethral incontinence

Extra-urethral incontinence occurs when the distal end of the ureter opens into a place other than the bladder, such as the rectum or perineum. A fistula – a passageway connecting the bladder to the bowel, resulting from trauma or infection following surgery – will also cause extra-urethral incontinence. Patients with extra-urethral incontinence need to be referred for surgery.

Functional incontinence

Functional incontinence is caused by problems of mobility and dexterity. Patients may find it difficult to reach the toilet in time because of physical and environmental factors. Functional incontinence should be treated by improving the patient's environment, by social care and aids, and by adaptations of lifestyle and clothing.

Follow-up treatment

At the end of the treatment session, it is helpful to make a list of questions to ask the patient when he attends for his next treatment. The progression in the number of repetitions and increase in hold time of PFMEs will depend on the results of another digital rectal assessment to ascertain the strength and endurance of the PFMs.

Treatment outcomes

Treatment aims to achieve urinary control, continence and confidence by conservative measures. However, it is not always possible to gain this outcome and patients may need help with managing their condition. It is important to set realistic goals.

Prevention of incontinence

Most clinicians who treat women with pelvic floor exercises believe that preventative exercises are beneficial. Many keep-fit classes for women include PFMEs. There are no trials concerning preventative pelvic floor exercises for men or women. However, it seems reasonable to suppose that keeping the PFMs in good tone would be beneficial in order to maintain normal function.

Pads

All patients should have a full continence assessment before being given pads. Conservative treatment may prevent the need for pads. However, patients may wish to wear a pad for confidence while receiving therapy and some patients, who find no improvement with therapy, may wish to manage the problem themselves.

Pads are usually composed of three layers: a non-woven surface, absorbent wood-pulp or tissue paper, and a waterproof backing (Pomfret, 1996). The size and shape of pads varies. Men may need the help of continence advisors to select a pad that is comfortable, contains urine and odour, and is reasonably priced. Stretch pants may hold the pad in place (Figure 8.10). Men with PMD may wish to use a dribble collector (Figure 8.11). This specially designed pouch has a pocket for the penis and testicles. The specially designed adhesive backing fastens the collector to the inside of tightly fitting briefs.

In an evaluation of 36 all-in-one disposable shaped incontinence pads, Pettersson and Fader (2000) found that there were wide variations in cost and absorbency and that price was a poor indicator of performance.

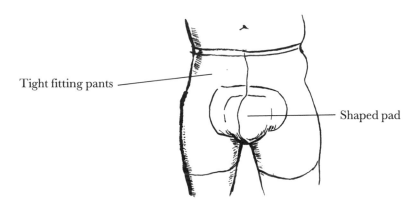

Tight fitting pants

Shaped pad

Figure 8.10 Shaped incontinence pad.

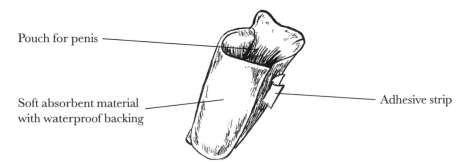

Pouch for penis

Soft absorbent material with waterproof backing

Adhesive strip

Figure 8.11 Dribble pouch.

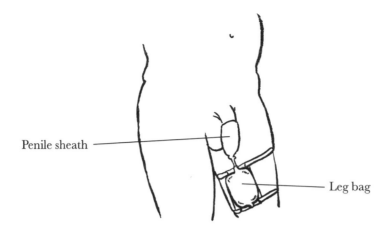

Figure 8.12 Sheath and leg bag.

From 192 recruits in 37 residential nursing homes, participants and carers indicated that a successful product needed to be able to contain urine without leaking and to have tabs for ease of opening and resealing.

In the Association for Continence Advice (ACA) Survey of Patients for the National Care Audit, 1998/9 (ACA, 2000), from 1915 men and women with incontinence, 25% of men used disposable pads, 6% of men used re-usable pads, 28% of men used a urisheath (sheath and drainage system) and only 7% of men managed their bladder problems with pelvic floor muscle exercises (ACA, 2000).

Appliances

All patients should have a full continence assessment before being given appliances. Conservative therapy can be given with the sheath and leg bag in place (Figure 8.12). Continence advisors are skilled at fitting the correct size of sheath which allows for changes in penis size. Some sheaths adhere to the penis whereas others have waist bands and groin straps (Pomfret, 1996). Skin care is paramount.

Skin care

Incontinence dermatitis is caused by a rise in the pH of the skin, increased permeability, increased hydration, attack by faecal enzymes, the action of certain skin preparations and the use of urine containment products (Le Lievre, 1999). The skin of men with incontinence dermatitis and urinary incontinence should be cared for as shown in Table 8.5.

Table 8.5 Care of the skin for incontinent patients

Avoid soaps and detergents which wash away protective oils
Wash in warm water alone or minimal amount of mild unperfumed soap
Avoid high temperature baths
Avoid soaking in the bath
Avoid talcum powder
Use only creams which contain high quantities of zinc
Pat skin completely dry and avoid vigorous rubbing
Use pads with superabsorbency which separates the urine from the skin
Check for latex allergy for men with sheaths and catheters
Avoid plastic pants and sheets which cause sweating

Intermittent self-catheterisation

Clean intermittent self-catheterisation (CISC) is used for men who are unable to empty their bladder completely by normal voiding. Men in this category include spinal injury patients and those with outflow obstruction.

Plastic catheters used for CISC fall into three groups:

- catheters requiring lubrication prior to insertion
- those with a hydrophilic coating, which when activated by water, provide a lubricated smooth surface for single use
- self-lubricated, silicone coated catheters for single use.

Other considerations are the position and smoothness of the drainage eyes in order to reduce the risk of urethral trauma. Patient preference will be influenced by convenience, ease of insertion, ease of removal and cost.

Artificial urinary sphincter

The artificial urinary sphincter is implanted surgically for patients with incontinence which has not responded to conservative treatment. It consists of a cuff round the urethra, a reservoir implanted in the abdomen, and a pump implanted in the scrotum (see Figure 8.13). To commence micturition, the scrotal pump is squeezed several times to transfer fluid from the urethral cuff into the abdominal reservoir. The cuff is automatically re-inflated after 2–3 min. In response to increased intra-abdominal pressure, additional fluid flows into the cuff to give extra intra-urethral pressure. The operation of this device needs good manual dexterity. The associated risks are mechanical failure, rejection and erosion through the urethra (Denning, 1996).

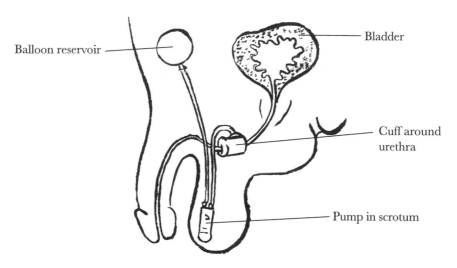

Figure 8.13 Artificial urinary sphincter.

Penile clamp

The penile clamp is still being used by some men to control their incontinence. Improperly used, the clamp may cause pressure necrosis to the penis and is therefore not usually recommended as a treatment option.

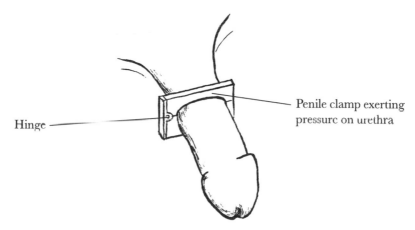

Figure 8.14 Penile clamp.

Interdisciplinary collaboration

For best practice, physiotherapists, continence advisors, urology nurses, urologists and GPs need to collaborate and provide an interdisciplinary service for male patients with LUTS.

In 1998 a consensus forum of key UK representatives from nurses and physiotherapists working in the specialised field of continence compiled a bipartite statement identifying the collaboration between the two professions (ICCC, 1998). A need to establish a working party to define core competencies and develop mutual education needs was identified. This collaboration was seen as an important breakthrough in the mutual understanding and roles of the two professions and serves as a basis for future networking for the benefit of the patient.

For interdisciplinary working to be successful it is essential that all disciplines are involved in free discussion and careful audit of the service (Haslam, 1996). Haslam stated that physiotherapists working as specialists in the field of incontinence had referred patients to the district nurse, occupational therapist, psychologist, dietician, GP, continence advisor, gynaecologist, urologist and community physiotherapist. Collaborative exchanges on patient care must be the model for the future. A continence service should include referral from any member of the interdisciplinary team and include self-referral. In conjunction with the wishes of the patient access should be available to any of the team who are specialised in male continence care. The network of team members is shown in Table 8.6.

Table 8.6 The interdisciplinary team involved in a continence service

Continence advisor
Nurse
Health visitor
Physiotherapist
Occupational therapist
Dietician
Social worker
Urologist
Geriatrician
Neurologist
General practitioner
Consultant in rehabilitation
Psychiatrist
Clinical psychologist
Coloproctologist
Gastroenterologist
Supplies staff
Voluntary bodies
Users and carers

The shared-care model provides a good example of how medical specialists and allied health professionals can work together to provide comprehensive healthcare of a high standard (Halloran, 1991).

Research opportunities

The challenge for professionals will be the integration of clinical evidence into practice and promoting and implementing prevention strategies. More research is needed to supplement these initiatives (Consensus Statement, 1997).

Suggestions for future research

Further research could take the form of qualitative studies in order to gain more detailed knowledge of the current treatment for men with LUTS, or it could take the form of quantitative trials by adding to the five existing RCTs (Paterson *et al*, 1997; Van Kampen *et al*, 1998; Moore *et al*, 1999 Bales *et al*, 2000, Porru *et al*, 2001). Collaborative multicentre studies could involve input from many urologists, nurses and physiotherapists in order to justify the current treatments for men with LUTS.

Qualitative research could take the form of focus groups or in-depth interviews of urologists, nurses, physiotherapists and patients, to identify the training needs of physiotherapists and nurses in this field. Specialised training could be provided to meet professional competencies.

The RCTs could explore the following topics:

- The optimum number, frequency and strength of PFM repetitions for the effective treatment of men with LUTS.
- The optimum position for performing PFMEs.
- The use of 'the knack' for patients with stress incontinence.
- The optimum time to begin pre-prostatectomy exercises.
- The use of immediate post-prostatectomy exercises (gently contracting on the catheter).
- A comparison of rectal and surface EMG biofeedback in men.
- The type, parameters and intensity of electrical stimulation for stress and urge incontinence in men.
- The behavioural and lifestyle changes for men with LUTS.

Case studies: questions and answers

1) A post-prostatectomy patient complains of leakage since his operation.

Q. How would you differentiate between:
(a) urge incontinence
(b) stress incontinence
(c) PMD
(d) overflow.
A. A frequency/volume (F/V) chart would show the number of voids, the amount voided, the amount of intake and output, the type of fluid drunk and the number of leaks of urine day and night. If there are nine or more voids per 24 h (normal about seven) and more than three voids at night, the patient may be suffering from frequency, urgency, urge incontinence and nocturia and may develop a low compliance bladder. From the F/V chart it can be determined if the patient is drinking excessively (normal intake is 1000–1500 ml per day) which would cause increased frequency. It is useful to monitor the urinary output. Urodynamics is a more invasive way of diagnosing stress or urge incontinence. The patient should be asked if his stream is reduced or if he is suffering from hesitancy and intermittency in case he has blockage from a stricture. Stress incontinence post-prostatectomy may be described subjectively as uncontrolled spurts of urine during activities which increase the intra-abdominal pressure. PMD (diagnosed subjectively) is leakage after micturition has been completed and the patient moves away from the bathroom. PMD should be distinguished from terminal dribble which is a dribble at the end of micturition.

2) A patient complains of increased urgency and frequency for three months. He has noticed some blood in his urine

Q. What are the possible diagnoses?
A. This patient could be suffering from a bladder infection, urethritis or bladder cancer. He would need a urine culture and antibiotics. If he has had a recent prostatectomy he may suffer with haematuria. Haematuria is also a sign of bladder cancer. He would need referring to a urologist for a cystoscopy to determine the problem.

3) A patient complains of increased problems of poor stream and difficulty initiating the stream. Recently he has been suffering from severe urge incontinence.

Q. How would you treat this patient?
A. The patient presents with increasing symptoms of obstruction. In addition he has developed symptoms of an unstable bladder. He would need referral to a urologist who would perform a digital rectal examination to exclude prostate cancer, and send the patient for uroflowmetry, an ultrasound scan to eliminate retention, and a blood test for prostate specific antigen (PSA). If the urologist diagnoses BPH, the patient may be treated with medication such as alpha-blockers to relax the bladder neck or 5-alpha reductase inhibitors to decrease the size of the prostate. The patient may be referred back to the therapist for treatment of the unstable bladder. The therapist could then give the patient PFMEs with biofeedback, teach urge suppression techniques, and provide advice on fluid adjustment.

4) A young man is sent to the GP by his partner to be treated for his severe urgency.

Q. What could be the possible causes of his urgency?
A. He may be suffering from sensory urgency due to:
(a) a high caffeine intake
(b) a high alcoholic intake
(c) urethritis
(d) cystitis
He may be suffering from motor urgency due to:
(a) idiopathic overactive bladder
(b) detrusor hyperreflexia resulting from a neurological condition

5) A patient is sent to you with PMD.

Q. What advice would you give him?
A. Initially, the patient could be taught to perform bulbar urethral massage after voiding. He should also be taught PFMEs in order to strengthen the bulbocavernosus muscle, which eliminates the last few drops of urine. He should be taught to contract his pelvic floor after he has completed micturition with a 'squeeze out' contraction.

Summary

Frequency, nocturia, urgency, urge incontinence, stress incontinence, PMD and post-prostatectomy incontinence can be treated conservatively. Treatment modalities include PFMEs, biofeedback, electrical treatment, lifestyle changes and bladder retraining.

Treatment progression is patient specific and dependent on ongoing assessment.

CHAPTER 9

Medication

Key points

- Medication may be prescribed for overactive bladder, nocturnal enuresis, BPH and prostate cancer.
- Some medication has an adverse effect on lower urinary tract function.
- Some medication changes the colour of the urine.

Pharmacotherapy for the overactive bladder

Pharmacotherapy can be used in the management of detrusor overactivity to reduce involuntary detrusor contractions and increase functional bladder capacity. Antimuscarinic drug therapy blocks the muscarinic receptors within the detrusor muscle that mediate detrusor contraction in normal men. Unwanted systemic effects of such drugs include dry mouth due to the inhibition of salivary secretion, blurring of near vision (cycloplegia), tachycardia and inhibition of gut motility leading to constipation (Wein, 1997). Bladder contractility is decreased and the bladder sphincter smooth muscle tone increased. Urinary retention may be a further unwanted side-effect. The most commonly used drugs in use at present in the UK are oxybutynin hydrochloride (Ditropan), tolterodine tartrate (Detrusitol) and imipramine (Tofranil). Tolterodine has the advantage of fewer side-effects. Dose titration is essential and patients should be advised that achieving the correct dose may require several visits to the clinician (McGuire and O'Connell, 1995). Drug therapy reduces detrusor instability but does not usually eliminate it (McGuire and O'Connell, 1995). Therefore, pharmacotherapy should be used in conjunction with bladder training and pelvic floor exercises in cases of moderate and severe urgency and urge incontinence.

Oxybutynin hydrochloride

Oxybutynin hydrochloride (Ditropan) is a tertiary amine with powerful anticholinergic (antimuscarinic), local anaesthetic and smooth muscle relaxation actions. The side-effects include dry mouth, reflux oesophagitis, dry skin, constipation and visual accommodation difficulties. Anticholinergic drugs are contraindicated in certain types of glaucoma. The starting dose is usually 2.5 mg daily and should be increased to 2.5 mg four times daily depending on the benefits and side-effects experienced.

Tolterodine tartrate

Tolterodine tartrate (Detrusitol) is a powerful antimuscarinic receptor antagonist with selectivity for the bladder rather than the salivary glands. Its tolerability and side-effect profile is generally favourable and somewhat better than that of oxybutynin (Abrams et al, 1998a; Drutz et al, 1999; Malone-Lee, 2000). The side-effects of tolterodine include dry mouth, dyspepsia, constipation and reduced lacrimation, but these anticholinergic effects have been found to be less than those experienced with oxybutynin. The most common side-effect is a dry mouth which occurs in 10% of patients (Abrams et al, 1998a). The recommended dose of 2 mg twice a day is equivalent in efficacy to oxybutynin at a dose of 5 mg twice a day or three times a day) (Malone-Lee, 2000).

Imipramine

Imipramine (Tofranil) is a tricyclic antidepressant which has anticholinergic, alpha-antagonistic, antihistamine, anti 5-HT and possible antidiuretic properties. It may be used in conjunction with oxybutynin in low doses. It is not licensed for use for an overactive bladder in the UK. It may help nocturnal enuresis. The side-effects of dry mouth, reflux oesophagitis, dry skin and visual accommodation difficulties are milder than those from oxybutynin. However, the elderly may experience postural instability and drowsiness. It has the potential to cause cardiac arrhythmias. It may help co-existing stress incontinence because of its alpha-adrenergic profile but it is not licensed for this use in the UK. The recommended dose is a single dose of between 10 mg and 25 mg at night (Castleden et al, 1986). An extra dose may be prescribed for those patients with troublesome daytime symptoms.

Other less commonly used drugs

There are a number of drugs, less commonly used than oxybutynin, tolterodine and imipramine, which may be used to treat the unstable bladder. Propiverine hydrochloride (Detrunorm) is an antimuscarinic agent with calcium blocking properties. It appears to be as effective as oxybutynin with less of the side-effects. The dosage of 15 mg twice daily can be increased to 15 mg three times daily or 15 mg four times daily (Halaska *et al*, 1994). Propantheline (Probanthine) is a quarternary ammonium compound, which is is not easily absorbed from the gastrointestinal tract. It is unlicensed for use for patients with an overactive bladder but was the standard drug until the introduction of oxybutynin. Flavoxate hydrochloride (Urispas) is a drug with antispasmodic and smooth muscle relaxation properties. Its efficacy is not established (Chapple *et al*, 1990). It has fewer side-effects than other drugs for an overactive bladder but very occasionally can cause nausea and vomiting.

Pharmacotherapy for nocturnal enuresis

Antidiuretic hormone analogues, such as the synthetic vasopressin desmopressin acetate (1-deamino-8-D-arginine vasopressin, DDAVP), cause decrease in urine production. Success rates of 75% have been reported in adult sufferers (Ramsden *et al*, 1982). DDAVP is available in both tablet form and nasal spray. Side-effects include headaches, abdominal pain, nasal stuffiness and epistaxis (nose bleed). Care must be taken in those with cardiac disease as DDAVP can provoke significant intravascular fluid overload.

Medication which may have an adverse effect on lower urinary tract function

Certain groups of drugs may have an adverse effect on the urinary system, especially in elderly people (Wagg and Malone-Lee, 1999).

Diuretics

Diuretics, such as theophylline which is used for asthma and the stimulant caffeine, increase urinary frequency and may cause urgency and urge incontinence in some men. Caffeine is sometimes added to medication to combat the side-effect of drowsiness that the drug produces.

Calcium-channel antagonists

This group of medication, which includes verapamil and amlodipine, may cause polyuria as a result of mobilisation of fluid from the extremities.

Non-steroidal anti-inflammatory drugs

These common medications, including ibuprofen and diclofenac, may cause salt and water retention.

Sedative medication

Sleeping tablets such as benzodiazepines (diazepam) and neuroleptics (chlorpromazine) may exacerbate existing urinary problems.

Anticholinergics

Anticholinergics such as antihistamines (terfenadine), antispasmodics (propantheline) antipsychotics (chlorpromazine) and drugs for Parkinson's disease (levodopa), may cause confusion in elderly people or urinary retention. They can exacerbate existing urinary problems.

Medication which reduces the size of the prostate gland

Drug therapy using 5-alpha reductase inhibitors decreases the size of the prostate by inhibiting the enzyme necessary for testosterone metabolism. Finasteride (Proscar) is a 5-alpha reductase inhibitor and is used to treat urethral blockage from benign prostatic hypertrophy (BPH). If the medication is withdrawn, the prostate gland will return to pre-treatment size or rebound with an increase in size. Finasteride acts by androgen deprivation and may be responsible for loss of libido in some men.

An extract from the berries of the American dwarf saw palmetto plant *Serenoa repens* is used to block 5-alpha reductase, thereby reducing the size of the prostate gland. From a systematic review of 18 randomised controlled trials, evidence suggested that *Serenoa repens* improved urological symptoms and urinary flow (Wilt *et al*, 1998). When compared to finasteride, *Serenoa repens* produced similar improvement in LUTS with fewer adverse effects. However, its long-term effectiveness remains unknown.

Medication which relaxes the smooth muscle of the bladder neck

Alpha-adrenoreceptor antagonists (alfuzosin, doxazosin) are alpha-block-ers which can be used for symptoms of obstruction because of their relax-ant effect on the prostate and internal urethral sphincter. Alpha-blockers such as prazosin hydrochloride (Hypovaze), doxazosin mesylate (Cardura) and alfazosin relax the smooth muscle of the bladder neck. The most frequently used alpha-blocker is prazosin hydrochloride which improves urinary flow rate and reduces day and night frequency. The medication may also have an effect on the intestinal smooth muscle resulting in constipation. Patients are warned they may have a retrograde ejaculation. These alpha-blockers may cause side-effects of dry mouth, sedation, dizziness, drowsiness, tachycardia and palpitations.

Medication for prostate cancer

Endocrine therapy includes gonadotrophin releasing hormone antagonists such as GnRHa (goserelin) and leuprorelin acetate or anti-androgen drug treatment (cyproterone acetate) as a treatment for prostate cancer. Side-effects include gynaecomastia, loss of libido and erectile dysfunction.

Medication for hypocontractile bladder

Cholinergic agonists such as carbachol and bethanechol can enhance detrusor contractions during micturition provided the problem is not too severe. Their use is limited because of their lack of efficacy.

Change in colour of the urine

Some medication and foods will change the colour of urine; some examples are given in Table 9.1.

Table 9.1. Changes in colour of urine

Medication or food	Resulting colour
Vitamin B	Yellow
Gantrisin (urinary antiseptic)	Red
Pyridium (urinary antiseptic)	Red
Nitrofurantoin (used for UTIs)	Brown
Beetroot	Pink
Asparagus	Yellow

Summary

Antimuscarinic drug therapy may be prescribed for detrusor overactivity. Antidiuretic hormone analogues may be prescribed for nocturnal enuresis. Drug therapy using 5-alpha reductase inhibitors reduce the size of the prostate, and alpha-blockers relax the smooth muscle of the bladder neck.

Endocrine therapy or anti-androgen drug treatment may be prescribed for prostate cancer.

Certain groups of drugs such as diuretics, calcium-channel antagonists, non-steroidal anti-inflammatory drugs, sedative medication, sleeping tablets and anticholinergics may have an adverse effect on lower urinary tract function especially in elderly people.

CHAPTER 10

Erectile dysfunction

Key points

- Over 152 million men worldwide suffer from erectile dysfunction.
- Risk factors are psychogenic, vasculogenic, neurogenic, endocrinologic, diabetic, drug-related, trauma-related and poor pelvic floor musculature.
- Erection may be classified as reflexogenic, psychogenic or nocturnal.
- The phases of erection are flaccidity, filling phase, tumescence, full erection, rigidity and detumescence.

Definition

Erectile dysfunction (ED) was defined by a National Institutes of Health Consensus Development Conference (NIH, 1993) as 'the inability to achieve or maintain an erection sufficient for satisfactory sexual performance'.

Prevalence

An estimated 152 million men worldwide suffered from erectile dysfunction in 1995 and this figure was projected to rise to 322 million men worldwide in 2025 (Aytac *et al*, 1999). Feldman *et al* (1994) found the problem was strongly age-related. They found that the probable prevalence of complete or partial erectile dysfunction rose from 40% in 50 year olds to 66% in 70 year olds. However, Lewis and Mills (1999) stated that age-related diseases may be the risk factors for erectile dysfunction rather than age itself. With increased life expectancy and a growing population, the number of men with erectile dysfunction will continue to increase.

The increased public awareness of the condition, due to the availability of sildenafil (Viagra), will result in a greater number of men seeking treatment. Sildenafil, however, produces adverse effects of headache, flushing, dyspepsia, nasal congestion, urinary tract infection, visual effects, diarrhoea and dizziness (Boolell *et al*, 1996). If it is taken more than once daily, back and leg aches, nausea, vomiting and diarrhoea have occurred (Colpo, 1998). It is absolutely contra-indicated for patients using any form of organic nitrates (Albaugh and Lewis, 1999).

Severity

There are varying degrees of erectile dysfunction; see Table 10.1

Table 10.1 Severity of erectile dysfunction (Albaugh and Lewis, 1999)

Severity	Satisfactory erection attempts out of 10
Mild	7–8
Moderate	4–6
Severe	0–3

Risk factors

Risk factors for erectile dysfunction include (Feldman *et al*, 1994):

- vascular insufficiency
- hormonal abnormalities
- interruption of the neural pathways
- psychogenic factors.

Also, Lewis and Mills (1999) list 332 prescription drugs that have been associated with erectile dysfunction. These include psychotrophic drugs, cardiovascular drugs, histamine-2-receptor antagonists, hormones, anticholinergics and certain cytotoxic agents. Another risk factor is diabetes mellitus; as many as 50% of men with diabetes may suffer from erectile dysfunction (Benet and Melman, 1995).

Other risk factors include accidental trauma, trauma from surgery and radiation therapy (Lewis and Mills, 1999). Lifestyle-related factors include cigarette smoking (Condra *et al*, 1986; Shabsigh *et al*, 1991; Butler *et al*, 1994; Mannino *et al*, 1994; Bortolotti *et al*, 1997; Jeremy and Mikhailidis, 1998; Tan and Philip, 1999; Dorey, 2001a), chronic obstructive lung disease, alcohol abuse (Gambert, 1997; O'Farrell *et al*, 1998; Tan and Philip, 1999), drug abuse (Benet and Melman, 1995); bicycling (Goodson, 1981; Amarenco *et al*, 1987; Solomon and Cappa, 1987; Desai and Gingell, 1989; Mellion, 1991; Andersen and Bovim, 1997; Nayal *et al*, 1999) and horse riding (Albaugh and Lewis, 1999).

Psychological causes

Erectile dysfunction always has a psychological component in addition to the underlying cause (Intili and Nier, 1998). In a pilot study of 15 men Intili and Nier (1998) found a link between erectile dysfunction and depression, and also between erectile dysfunction and low self-esteem.

The psychological causes of erectile dysfunction have been classified as religious orthodoxy, obsessive-compulsive personality, gender identity, sexual phobias, widower's syndrome, fear of pregnancy, marital conflict, depression, lack of attraction to partner, fear of closeness, poor body image and concern over ageing (LoPiccolo, 1986). The International Society of Impotence Research (ISIR) divide psychogenic factors into 'generalised type', which includes 'generalised unresponsiveness' and 'generalised inhibition'; and 'situational type', which includes 'partner related', 'performance related' and 'psychological distress or adjustment related' (Lizza and Rosen, 1999) (see Table 10.2).

Table 10.2 Classification of the psychological causes of erectile dysfunction

LoPiccolo (LoPiccolo, 1986)	ISIR classification (Lizza and Rosen, 1999)
Psychological causes	**Psychogenic factors**
Religious orthodoxy	**Generalised type**
Obsessive-compulsive personality	Generalised unresponsiveness
Gender identity	Generalised inhibition
Sexual phobias	
Widower's syndrome	**Situational type**
Fear of pregnancy	Partner related
Marital conflict	Performance related
Depression	Psychological distress or adjustment related
Lack of attraction to partner	
Fear of closeness	
Poor body image	
Concern over ageing	

There is a growing opinion that weakness of the bulbocavernosus and ischiocavernosus muscles may be a risk factor for erectile dysfunction (Claes and Baert, 1993; Colpi *et al*, 1994; Ballard, 1997; Van Kampen, 1998; Colpi *et al*, 1999; Mamberti-Dias *et al*, 1999). The risk factors for erectile dysfunction are summarised in Table 10.3.

Table 10.3 Risk factors for erectile dysfunction

Psychogenic	Marital conflict, depression, poor body image, performance related
Vasculogenic	Arteriogenic and venogenic
Neurogenic	Spinal cord trauma, multiple sclerosis, spinal tumours
Endocrinologic	Hormonal deficiency, eugonadotrophic hypogonadism
Diabetic	Linked to peripheral neuropathy, hypertension and renal failure
Drug-related	Antihypertensives, psychotropics, hormonal agents
Surgical trauma	Transurethral prostatectomy, radical prostatectomy, other pelvic surgery
Lifestyle related	Blunt trauma to the perineum, cigarette smoking, drug abuse, alcohol abuse
Weak perineal musculature	Lack of use? ageing?

Anatomy of the penis

The penis consists of three cylindrical erectile bodies: dorsally, the two corpora cavernosa communicate with each other for three-quarters of their length and ventrally the corpus spongiosum surrounds the penile portion of the urethra. The proximal end of the corpus spongiosum forms a bulb attached to the urogenital diaphragm and at the distal end expands to form the glans penis (Kirby *et al*, 1999) (Figures 10.1 and 10.2).

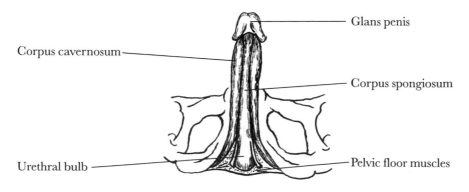

Figure 10.1 Anatomy of the penis.

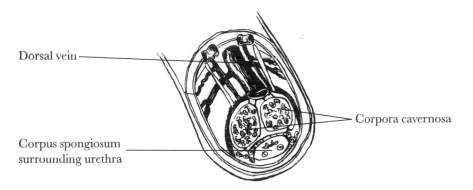

Figure 10.2 Cross-section of the penis.

Muscles associated with penile rigidity

The muscles influencing penile rigidity are the ischiocavernosus and the bulbocavernosus (bulbospongiosus) muscles. The ischiocavernosus muscle is a paired muscle which arises from the medial aspect of the ischial tuberosity and inserts into the medial and inferior surface of the corporal bodies. The bulbocavernosus muscle originates from the central perineal tendon and attaches to the dorsal surface of the corpus spongiosum. Contractions of the ischiocavernosus muscles produce an increase in the intracavernous pressure. Rhythmic contraction of the bulbocavernosus muscle propels the semen down the urethra resulting in ejaculation. Following micturition, the bulbocavernosus muscle helps to empty the last few drops of urine. Both muscles are supplied by the perineal branch of the pudendal nerve (S3–4) (see Figure 10.3).

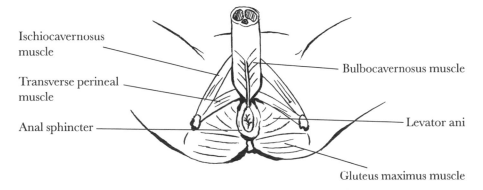

Figure 10.3 Male superficial pelvic floor muscles.

Houston's muscles (compressor venous dorsalis) are often mistaken for the bulbocavernosus muscles. They compress the deep dorsal veins and prevent venous reflux. Contractions of the ischiocavernosus and bulbo-cavernosus muscles force blood into the anterior part of the penis and the contraction of Houston's muscles block venous drainage (Lavoisier *et al*, 1988; Poirier and Charpy, 1901; Wespes *et al*, 1990).

Physiology of penile erection

Neurophysiologically, erection can be classified into three types (Brock and Lue, 1993):

Reflexogenic erection

Reflexogenic erection originates from tactile stimulation to the genitalia. Impulses reach the spinal erection centre (S2–4 and T10–L2) and some follow the ascending tract culminating in sensory perception, while others activate the autonomic nuclei of the efferent nerves which induce the erection process.

Psychogenic erection

Psychogenic erection originates from audiovisual stimuli or fantasy. Signals descend to the spinal erection centre to activate the erection process.

Nocturnal erection

Nocturnal erection occurs mostly during the rapid eye movement stage of sleep. Most men experience 3–5 erections lasting up to 30 min in a normal night's sleep (Fisher *et al*, 1965). Central impulses descend the spinal cord (through an unknown mechanism) to activate the erection process.

Mechanism of erection

Penile erection occurs following a series of integrated vascular events culminating in the accumulation of blood under pressure and end-organ rigidity (Moncada Iribarren and Sáenz de Tejada, 1999). The vascular process of erection can be divided into five phases:

* **Flaccidity:** A state of low flow of blood and low pressure exists in the penis.

- **Latent or filling phase:** When the erection mechanism is initiated by any stimulus, the penile smooth arterial muscle relaxes and the cavernosal and helicine arteries dilate enabling blood to flow into the lacunar spaces (see Figure 10.4).
- **Tumescence:** The venous outflow is reduced by the compression of the subtunical venules against the tunica albuginea (corporal veno-occlusive mechanism) causing the penis to expand and elongate but with a scant increase in intracavernous pressure.
- **Full erection:** The intracavernous pressure rapidly increases.
- **Rigidity:** The intracavernous pressure rises higher than the diastolic pressure and blood inflow occurs with the systolic phase of the pulse enabling complete rigidity to occur. Contraction or reflex contraction of the ischiocavernosus and bulbocavernosus muscles produces changes in the intracavernous pressure. No arterial flow occurs.

Flaccid state

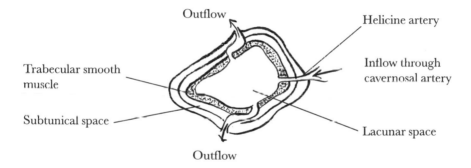

Erect State

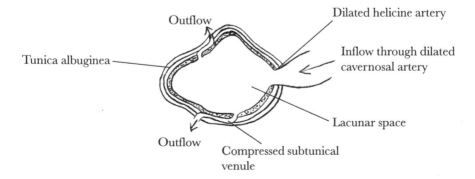

Figure 10.4 Veno-occlusive mechanism.

- **Detumescence:** Contraction of the penile smooth muscles and contraction of the penile arteries leads to a decrease of blood in the lacunar spaces and the contraction of the smooth trabecular muscle leads to a collapse of the lacunar spaces.

Mechanism of ejaculation

Ejaculation requires interaction of the sympathetic T10–L2, parasympathetic S2–4 and somatic nerves S2–4 and can occur independently of penile erection. Stimulation of the superior hypogastric or hypogastric nerves causes contraction of the bladder neck, seminal vesicles and ejaculatory ducts. Contraction of the periurethral and PFMs combined with intermittent relaxation of the external urinary sphincter and urogenital diaphragm allows ejaculation (Krane *et al*, 1989). The experience of orgasm is independent of sympathetic and parasympathetic activity but it does require an intact pudendal nerve (Mamberti-Dias *et al*, 1999).

Summary

Erectile dysfunction may be classified as mild, moderate or severe according to the proportion of satisfactory erection attempts.

Risk factors for erectile dysfunction may be classified as psychogenic, vasculogenic, neurogenic, endocrinologic, diabetic, drug-related, trauma-related and poor pelvic floor musculature.

CHAPTER 11

Conservative treatment for erectile dysfunction

Key points

* Ischiocavernosus and bulbocavernosus muscle activity increase penile rigidity in the tumescent penis.
* Pelvic floor muscle efficiency is higher in potent than impotent men.
* Pelvic floor muscle efficiency reduces with age in impotent men.
* PFMEs could be practised simultaneously for erectile dysfunction and incontinence.

Literature search

A literature search by Dorey (2000c–e) revealed only 16 clinical trials detailing conservative treatment for erectile dysfunction (ED). Fourteen trials met the broad selection criteria and were included in this review. The selection criteria included those trials which reported the results of physical therapy interventions for men with erectile dysfunction with clinically relevant and reliable outcome measures. One study used subcutaneous nerve electrical stimulation with a subcutaneous penile electrode which was beyond the scope of physiotherapists and therefore excluded in this review, but the results were tabulated because of the close relationship with the literature review (Shafik, 1996). Three clinical trials which monitored activity in the ischiocavernosus muscle using needle EMG, an invasive method of biofeedback (Lavoisier et al, 1986; Claes and Baert, 1993; Claes et al, 1995) and one trial which measured pressure from a transducer in the corpus cavernosum were included in the review for completeness (Lavoisier et al, 1986). One abstract from Russia (Karpukhin and Bogomol'nyi, 1999) revealed that the use of shock-wave massage, mud applications and local vacuum magnetotherapy stimulated copulative function.

Only four trials included a control group (Colpi *et al*, 1994; Stief *et al*, 1996; Aydin *et al*, 1997; Colpi *et al*, 1999) and only one used randomisation (Aydin *et al*, 1997).

From the literature review, a table was compiled of the conservative treatment for erectile dysfunction (Table 11.1).

Table 11.1 Part 1 Conservative treatment for erectile dysfunction

Author/design	Subjects	Method	Parameters	Outcomes
Claes & Bart 1993 Belgium *British Journal of Urology* Randomised No control	150 ED & VL age 23–64 median 48.7 Group 1 72 surgery Group 2 78 PFMEs	Group 1 Surgery deep dorsal vein Group 2 Information Self digital ICM 5 weekly PFMEs & ICM's Home ex pr. sit & st. Dig. eval. initially 4 & 12 months 40mg papaverine +EMG max contract ICM's	EMG needle ICM	Group 1 at 4 months 44 (61%) cured 17 (23.6%) improved 11 (15.2%) failed Group 2 at 4 months 36 (46%) cured 22 (28%) improved 20 (25.6%) failed Group 1 at 12 months 30 (42%) cured 23 (32% improved Group 2 at 12 months 33 (42%) cured 24 (31 %) improved 45 (58%) refused surgery Subjective outcome
Lavoisier *et al* 1988 Canada *Journal of Urology* Not random No control	7 psych ED Age 28–50 mean 38.2	To record 1CP and ICM activity with nocturnal erections Penile cuff and Surface EMG	Surface EMG over 1CM	Over 300mmHg ICP triggered by ICM's Objective outcome measured by authors
Mamberti-Dias *et al* 1991 France *Sexologique* Not random No control	210 ED Mean 52.5 Some VL Some psychological	PFMEs & EMG & electrical stimulation sacral & penile or perineal electrode Visual stimulation & penile temperature 15 treatments	5 – 25HZ and then 50 – 400Hz Intermittent	111 (53%) cured 44 (21%) improved 55 (26%) failed 67% of patients attained 4/10 to 8/10 ISMR Subjective outcome
Colpi *et al* 1994 Italy *Journal of Endocrinology Invest* Not random Controlled	59 ED & YL Age 20–63 mean & median 39 Group 1 33 PFMEs+ BFB Group 2 26 Controls	30 of 59 DDV incision 30 of 59 Psychosexual therapy No info which? Group 1 PFMEs +BFB Group 2 Controls	No information on type of BFB	Group 1 21 (63%) out of 33 who did PFMEs cured or improved Group 2 4 (15%) out of 26 no PFME cured or improved 9 refused surgery Subjective outcome

Table 11.1 Part 2 Review of the literature: pelvic floor exercises for erectile dysfunction

Author/design	Subjects	Method	Parameters	Outcomes
Lavoisier et al 1986 Canada Journal of Urology Not random No control	9 ED (no VL) Age 29–65 mean 41.8.	Artificial saline erection + maximal ICM contractions needle EMG + transducer corpus cavernosum	N/A	Increases in ICP in phase with greater ICM activity Significant (p<0.01) Objective outcome measured by authors
Stief et al 1996 Germany Urologe A Not random Controlled	22 ED vasoactive non-responders	Transcutaneous electrical stim. to smooth muscle corpus cavernosum	Low frequency symmetrical trapezoidal 100–2000μsecs, approx 12mA 0.5 secs rise 5 secs stimulation 0.5 secs rest alternating 10–20Hz and 20–35Hz	5 (23%) cured 3(13.60%) responded to vaso-active drugs 14 (63.6%) failed Subjective outcome
Derouet et al 1998 Germany European Urology Not random No control	48 ED	Transcutaneous electrical stimulation penile or perineal electrodes 20mins daily for 3 months	Bipolar, triangular DC-free pulse 85μs 30Hz 3 secs stimulation 6 secs rest 20–120mA	5 (10.4%) cured 20 (41.6% improved 23 (47.9%) failed including 10 drop outs Subjective outcome
Claes et al 1996a Belgium Journal of Urology Supplement Not random No control	178 ED Age 21–76 median 53.3	PFMEs and electrical stimulation No information on protocol	No information	47 (26%) cured 55 (31%) improved 47 (26%) failed including 19 drop outs Subjective outcome
Van Kampen et al 1998 Belgium PhD Thesis Katholieke Univesiteit Leuven Not random No control	51 ED various causes Age 25–64 mean 46	Patient education Role of ICM & BCM PFMEs short and long in lie sit and stand + BFB rectal pressure + 15 mins ES anal electrode or surface electrode once a week for 4 months 90 contractions daily home ex	Symmetrical biphasic low freq. 50Hz 200μsecs 6 secs stimulation 12 secs rest	24 (46% cured 12 (24%) improved 15 (31%) failed including 9 drop outs Subjective outcome

Table 11.1 Part 3 Conservative treatment for erectile dysfunction

Author/Design	Subjects	Method	Parameters	Outcomes
Claes *et al* 1995 Belgium *European Journal of Physical Medicine Rehabilitation* Not random No control	122 ED & VL Age 21–63 Median 49.5	Patient education role of ICM & BCM +PFM short & long +EMG BFB or manometric BFB +15 minutes ES rectal or surface electrode +home exercises 40 short 50 long Evaluation initially 4 & 12 months by needle EMG of ICM	Symmetrical biphasic low frequency 50Hz pulse 100μsecs 6 secs stimulation 12 secs rest maximum comfortable intensity	At 4 months 53 (43%) cured 37 (30%) improved 32 (26.2%) failed incl. 14 drop outs At 12 months 44 (36%) cured 41 (33.6%) improved 37 (30.3%) failed incl. 14 drop outs 65 (53.4%) patients refused surgery Subjective outcome
Schouman Lacroix 1991 France *Ann Urologique* Not random No control	20 ED Group 1 10 VL Group 2 10 Psychogenic	Both groups 10mg papaverine ES ICM & BCM surface electrodes + ES rectal electrode +PFMEs +EMG BFB position of sensors unknown 16 sessions in 8 weeks Eval. 6 months	No information	At 6 months Group 1 6 (60%) cured or improved 4 (40%) failed Group 2 5 (50%) cured or improved 5 (50%) failed including 1 drop out Subjective outcome
Kho *et al* 1999 Netherlands *International Journal of Impotence Research* Not random No control	16 ED	Acupuncture for 30 mins twice a week for 4 weeks using same 8 acupoints 30 mins ES to 4 acupoints Evaluation diary and partner's diary 4 weeks before Rx: 4 weeks Rx: 4 weeks after Rx:	Swiss constant current Doltron ESA 600 stimulator low frequency 5Hz and 10mA	2 (15%) improved 5 (31%) increased sexual activity Subjective outcome + partner's independent verification
Aydin et al 1997 Turkey *Scandinavian Journal of Urology and Nephrology* Randomised Controlled	60 ED no organic cause Group 1 15 men mean age 36.7±10.43 Group 2 16 men mean age 35.5±11.52 Group 3 15 men Group 4 14 men	Group 1 Electro-acpuncture 6 classic points Group 2 Hypnosis 3 days a month > once a month Group 3 Oral vitamin pill placebo Group 4 Placebo needle puncture non-classical points +	3Hz stimulation of direct current	Group 1 9 (60%) cured 6 (40%) failed Group 2 12 (75%) cured 4 (25%) failed Group 3 7 (47%) cured 8 (53%) failed Group 4 7 (47%) cured 8 (57%) failed (p=0.26625)

	Group 3 & 4 29 men mean age 36±11.38	electrostimulation Therapy twice a week for 6 weeks		Subjective outcome + partner's independent verification
Shafik 1996 Egypt *Andrologia* Not random No control	15 men ED age 32–55 mean 42.6	Cavernous nerve exposed through parapenile incision Electrical stimulation Bipolar platinum electrode implanted with subcutaneous receiver	10Hz and 60Hz	Electrical stimulation at 10Hz led to tumescence and increased intracavernous pressure (P<0.01) 60Hz led to full erection Objective outcomes by author
Colpi *et al* 1999 Italy *International Journal of Impotence Research* Not random Controlled	Group 1 76 potent men Age 18–35 mean 29.3±3.6 Group 2 97 men with ED Age 18–35 mean 28.1±4.1 Group 3 127 men with ED Age 36–50 mean 43.7±4.2 Group 4 90 men with ED Age 51–75 mean 58.3+5.5	Imitation of coital thrusts in side lying to increase rigidity of penis 24 maximal contractions 3 seconds hold and 6 secs rest EMG rectal probe 2 surface electrodes on perineum and antagonists 1 grounded electrode	N/A	Myoelectric activity of the perineum significantly higher in potent men compared to age matched impotent men Myoelectric activity of perineum significantly lower in men with ED over 50 compared to younger men with ED up to 35 and men up to 50 years Objective outcomes by authors

Treatment for different categories of erectile dysfunction

The literature review revealed that Claes and Baert (1993), Colpi *et al* (1994) and Claes *et al* (1995) treated only erectile dysfunction due to venous leakage with PFMEs, whereas Schouman and Lacroix (1991) split the sample into those men with erectile dysfunction due to venous leakage and those with a psychogenic cause. Van Kampen (1998) classified the type of erectile dysfunction into the categories of venous leakage, arteriogenic, venous leakage plus arteriogenic, psychogenic and unclassified, whereas Colpi *et al* (1999) categorised the aetiological factors as psychogenic, venogenic, arteriogenic, neurogenic, fibrosis, pharmaco-logic, endocrine and diabetic.

Trials were conducted in Canada, Belgium, France, Germany, Italy, The Netherlands and Turkey. There were no trials from the UK. It may be that health professionals in the UK were unwilling to explore this area because of reticence and a belief that psychogenic factors play a strong role. Taking our cultural differences into account, psychogenic factors may be different in British men.

Patient information

All treatments should start with patient education, including an explana-tion of the patient's condition and the treatment options available. It is helpful to use a model of the male pelvis complete with musculature in order to explain the anatomy and physiology. Only three erectile dysfunc-tion trials included patient education with emphasis on the pelvic anatomy, and the function and position of the ischiocavernosus muscles and bulbocavernosus muscles (Claes and Baert, 1993; Claes *et al*, 1996a; Van Kampen, 1998).

Pelvic floor muscle exercises

From the literature review, it appears that pelvic floor exercises have considerable merit as a treatment for erectile dysfunction for patients with venous leakage. They may also be useful for erectile dysfunction resulting from other causes such as poor musculature or a psychogenic origin. They are non-invasive, easy to perform, painless, cost effective, and free from drug side-effects. Pelvic floor exercises should be targeted at the ischiocavernosus and bulbocavernosus muscles.

Eight of the trials used pelvic floor muscle exercises (PFMEs) (Mamberti-Dias and Bonierbale-Branchereau, 1991; Schouman and Lacroix, 1991; Claes and Baert, 1993; Colpi *et al*, 1994, 1999; Claes *et al*, 1995, 1996a; Van Kampen, 1998). Claes and Baert (1993) used randomi-sation and compared a group performing PFMEs with a group undergo-ing surgery for erectile dysfunction. The literature review showed encouraging results from each of the ten studies using PFMEs for the treatment of erectile dysfunction (Dorey, 2000a–c). The results showed that maximal pelvic floor muscle work may aid penile rigidity, and cure or improve erectile dysfunction.

Patients performing PFMEs for urinary incontinence could combine a simultaneous training programme of PFMEs for erectile dysfunction.

Specific ischiocavernosus and bulbocavernosus muscle exercises

The method of performing PFMEs varied. In the study by Claes and Baert (1993), patients were also taught to tighten the ischiocavernosus muscles. In the study by Schouman and Lacroix (1991) patients were taught to tighten the ischiocavernosus and bulbocavernosus muscles while achieving rigidity with 10 mg of papaverine. However, in the study by Claes and Baert (1993) patients were injected with 40 mg papaverine to achieve penile rigidity and tested with needle EMG while contracting the ischiocavernosus muscle maximally.

In four trials, men were encouraged to perform specific ischiocavernosus and bulbocavernosus muscle exercises as opposed to just PFMEs (Schouman and Lacroix, 1991; Claes and Baert, 1993; Claes et al, 1993; Van Kampen, 1998). In four studies men performed ischiocavernosus and bulbocavernosus muscle exercises with an erect penis showing the need for exercising the specific muscles concerned with penile rigidity (Lavoisier et al, 1986; Schouman and Lacroix, 1991; Wespes et al, 1990; Colpi et al, 1999). Lavoisier et al (1986) showed that patients with erectile dysfunction but without venous occlusive dysfunction gained increased intracavernous pressure when asked to perform maximal voluntary contractions of the ischiocavernosus muscles with an artificially induced erection. They stated that this increase in intracavernous pressure would not have occurred if the cavernosus cavities were not completely engorged. This research indicated that men should be advised to use these muscles during coitus. During the thrust phase of coitus, the levator ani works synergically with the gluteus maximus muscle, obturator internus muscle and the other lateral hip rotators (Mamberti-Dias et al, 1999). This would pose a need for optimum muscular strength and endurance and a good level of cardiovascular fitness.

PFMEs to produce increase in intracavernous pressure

The trials by Lavoisier et al (1986) and Wespes et al (1990) demonstrated the increase in the intracavernous pressure during contractions of the ischiocavernosus and bulbocavernosus muscle in men with erectile dysfunction. Lavoisier et al (1986) showed an increase of between

100 mm Hg and 525 mm Hg (average 298 mm Hg) whereas Michal *et al* (1983) demonstrated only an increase in the intracavernous pressure of the tumescent penis of at least 100 mm Hg by pelvic floor contractions in healthy men. These three trials reflect laboratory conditions, whereas Meehan and Goldstein (1983) showed that during self-stimulation the intracavernous pressure increased to 10 times the arterial blood pressure. The ischiocavernosus muscle has clearly been shown to have a role in increasing the pressure in the tumescent penis, which links in with the work performed by Claes *et al* (1996b) who dissected the corpora cavernosa of 30 male cadavers and found that the area of the corpora cavernosum compressed by the ischiocavernosus muscle ranged from 35.6% to 55.9%.

PFMEs with biofeedback

Five trials used PFMEs with biofeedback in order to provide patient awareness and stimulate increased effort. Of these, two included biofeedback as the only other modality (Colpi *et al*, 1994, 1999), and three combined PFMEs with biofeedback and electrical stimulation (Schouman and Lacroix, 1991; Claes *et al*, 1995; Van Kampen, 1998). However, it was impossible to determine which modality has caused the effect when three modalities were used. Similar techniques have been used to treat urinary and faecal incontinence and other pelvic muscle dysfunctions (La Pera and Nicastro, 1996; Ballard, 1997; Mamberti-Dias *et al*, 1999).

La Pera and Nicastro (1996) used PFMEs, pressure biofeedback and electrical stimulation in a non-randomised and non-controlled trial of 18 patients aged 34 (range 20–52 years) to treat premature ejaculation. The results showed that 11 patients (61%) were cured as a result of PFM control. Lombardi (1999) also used electrical stimulation alternated with biofeedback for premature ejaculation (details unknown).

Biofeedback was obtained in a variety of ways; needle EMG, surface or rectal EMG, and manometric rectal pressure. Colpi *et al* (1999) in his successful study used perineal EMG to have 'kinesiologic clues of all the cloacal muscles'. Rectal manometry and rectal EMG would monitor the PFMs but perineal EMG would target the ischiocavernosus muscles, the muscles demonstrated to increase intracavernous pressure and therefore increase penile rigidity.

It was impossible to tell from the literature if biofeedback enhanced exercise performance or improved the effect of PFMEs. It seems reasonable to suppose that EMG to the ischiocavernosus muscles would monitor the muscles concerned with penile erection and intracavernous pressure increases rather than using biofeedback with a rectal pressure probe. Instead of using invasive needle EMG, muscle activity of the ischiocavernosus muscle and the bulbocavernosus muscle may be monitored by small surface EMG sensors.

Electrical stimulation for the treatment of erectile dysfunction

The parameters of electrical stimulation were given in six out of seven studies (Derouet *et al*, 1998; Mamberti-Dias and Bonierbale-Branchereau, 1991; Claes and Baert, 1993; Claes *et al*, 1995; Stief *et al*, 1996; Van Kampen, 1998).

When electrical stimulation was combined with PFMEs it was impossible to know which modality produced the effect. However, two trials used electrical stimulation alone. Derouet *et al* (1998) found electrical stimulation to the ischiocavernosus muscle produced only a 10.4% cure rate whereas Stief *et al* (1996) in a controlled trial explored transcutaneous electrical stimulation to the smooth muscle of the penile corpus cavernosum and effected a 23% cure rate. With penile electrodes, simultaneous stimulation of cavernosus smooth muscle tissue cannot be excluded from the study by Derouet *et al* (1988), even though the pulse protocol and parameters were designed for striated muscle. Whatever effect was achieved, both cure rates were low compared to the PFME trials. This endorsed the work by Berghmans *et al* (1998) who systematically reviewed treatment for female stress incontinence and stated that electrical stimulation may be no more effective than PFMEs alone but may be particularly appropriate to initiate a muscle contraction.

Acupuncture for the treatment of erectile dysfunction

Acupuncture may have a place in the treatment of erectile dysfunction, but the evidence is not very convincing. Only two papers using small samples were found. Both used electro-acupuncture. The study by Kho *et al* (1999) advised a further study and the study by Aydin *et al* (1997) found hypnosis superior to electro-acupuncture but also obtained good results from the controls. In the trial by Aydin *et al* (1997) one could argue that the needle puncture group received electrical stimulation and were therefore not true controls. However, in the vitamin placebo group seven patients were cured. As these patients had no organic cause, this may be due to the 'treatment effect' improving erectile function by relieving anxiety and mental stress. Psychological factors must have a role and be taken into account in the design of research studies.

Advice for patients with erectile dysfunction

Only one study indicated the advice given to the patients. Mamberti-Dias and Bonierbale-Branchereau (1991) gave advice concerning visual erotic stimulation and the ability to fantasise. Men with a psychological cause may also benefit from sex therapy, or it may be that all patients may benefit from this form of treatment. Men suffering from erectile dysfunction due to organic causes may have a psychosomatic overlay resulting from performance anxiety and the accompanying stress produced.

Mamberti-Dias *et al* (1999) stated that there must be an ischiocavernosus reflex similar to the bulbocavernosus reflex (pressure on the glans penis elicits a contraction of the bulbocavernosus muscles in a neurologically intact man) which can be triggered by a variation of pressure from 20 to 40 mm Hg on the glans penis. Mamberti-Dias *et al* (1999) showed various changes in vaginal pressure during coitus, with peaks at the vaginal entrance, the junction between the external third and internal two-thirds, with contact of the cervix, and at the beginning of withdrawal. They suggested slow rather than fast movement for maximum maintenance of rigidity, as slow movements generate higher intracavernous pressure. This links with the study by Lavoisier *et al* (1992) who hypothesised that during coitus, the glans penis was subjected to varying amounts of phasic pressure stimulation, which elicited reflex contractions of the ischiocavernosus muscles and increased penile rigidity.

Psychosexual issues

All the trials used a sample of heterosexual men. No study mentioned any cultural factors. The perceptions of sexual activity vary from one man to another and impact on the expectations and the subjective measurement of sexual performance. Not all men wish to practise penetrative sex. There were no studies which identified and addressed the difficulties and needs of homosexual men who practise anal intercourse. These factors underpin issues in the counselling of patients with erectile dysfunction.

Lifestyle changes

Patients may be advised that there are a number of ways to change their lifestyle in order to improve their health and well-being. These changes may help improve penile erection.

Alcohol

Excess intake of alcohol can lead to erectile difficulties (Gambert, 1997; Kosch *et al*, 1988; O'Farrell *et al*, 1998; Fabra and Porst, 1999; Tan and Philip, 1999; Wetterling *et al*, 1999). It may help to reduce the daily intake to two units of alcohol a day or less (one pint of beer or two small whiskies or two small glasses of wine).

The effect of alcohol on performance has been well known for generations. It was documented by William Shakespeare:

> *Porter*: Drink, sir, is a great provoker of three things.
> *Macduff*: What three things does drink especially provoke?
> *Porter*: Marry, sir, nose-painting, sleep and urine. Lechery, sir, it provokes and unprovokes; it provokes the desire but takes away the performance' (*Macbeth*)

Smoking

Smoking has been found to adversely affect the peripheral circulation and may produce erectile difficulties (Condra *et al*, 1986; Kosch *et al*, 1988; Shabsigh *et al*, 1991; Butler *et al*, 1994; Vidal Moreno *et al*, 1996; Melman and Gingell, 1999; Tan and Philip, 1999; Dorey, 2001d). Cessation of smoking may restore normal function (Mikhailidis *et al*, 1998). Data suggests that sexual dysfunction worsens as chronic obstructive lung disease worsens (Fletcher and Martin, 1982).

General fitness

Men can have erectile difficulties from being unfit, having high blood pressure and cardiopulmonary problems (Kosch *et al*, 1988; Butler *et al*, 1994; Pinnock *et al*, 1999). Fitness levels may be gradually increased by regular exercise such as walking every day, swimming, sport or by exercising in a gym at least twice a week.

Weight reduction

Obesity can put a strain on the heart and lead to high blood pressure which in turn can affect penile erection (Butler *et al*, 1994). Chung *et al*

(1999) found obesity in itself not to be a problem but it imposed a risk of vasculogenic erectile dysfunction from chronic vascular disease. Patients could be advised to change to a low fat diet, see a dietician or join a weight reduction group.

Cycling

It has been shown that long-distance cycling can restrict the circulation to the pelvic floor and the penis (Desai and Gingell, 1989). Nayal *et al* (1999) demonstrated that the penile oxygen values decreased during cycling. The saddle pressure from prolonged cycling may cause peripheral nerve compression and damage the pudendal nerve serving the penis (Amarenco *et al*, 1987; Mellion, 1991; Andersen and Bovim, 1997). A relationship between sexual dysfunction and bicycling resulting from vascular and neural compression may be more common than was formerly suspected (Solomon and Cappa, 1987). Patients should be advised to lift themselves off the saddle at regular intervals.

Number of treatments

No RCTs have been conducted on the optimum number of treatment sessions for PFMEs. In the literature reviewed, the amount of treatment varied from 5 to 20 treatment sessions, although some papers did not divulge this information.

In clinical practice, exercise regimes need to be patient specific. Therefore they are bound to be variable in number when patients are not in a research study.

Follow-up assessments

Colpi *et al* (1994) expected men to perform daily home exercises for 9 months as a realistic alternative to surgery. No trial mentioned a long-term follow-up or advised a maintenance programme for life, although Claes and Baert (1993), and Claes *et al* (1995) followed up subjects for 12 months with encouraging results. For those patients who have been cured or improved with PFMEs, it would be prudent to continue these simple exercises for life and avoid a return of erectile dysfunction, or surgery.

In the 14 trials reviewed, patients were assessed initially, and then between 3 months and 12 months.

Prevention of erectile dysfunction

Colpi et al (1999) monitored the strength of the perineal muscles by EMG in right side lying with the subjects imitating coital thrusts. They found that the perineal muscle contraction was significantly higher in potent men than age-matched impotent men; and that in impotent men over 51 years the perineal efficiency was significantly reduced. They concluded that ageing may affect voluntary contractile capacity because there is a tendency to a more sedentary lifestyle and to systemic pathologies, such as diabetes, hepatopathy, arteriosclerosis, and neuropathies which may cause decreases in muscle mass. PFMEs could be used to prevent or reverse muscle weakness caused by disuse and may delay the onset of some pathologies.

If the activity of the ischiocavernosus muscles increase penile rigidity, then weak musculature due to ageing could produce a decrease in penile rigidity and a serious reason for erectile dysfunction. This links in well with the work of Colpi et al (1999) who demonstrated that perineal muscle efficiency was decreased in patients suffering from erectile dysfunction and with ageing.

There were no publications describing preventative conservative treatment. But if the pelvic floor musculature is poor, and PFMEs can be demonstrated to relieve erectile dysfunction, then it seems reasonable to suppose that preventative muscle strengthening may help to prevent erectile dysfunction. The age old adage 'Use it or lose it' applies aptly to the pelvic floor musculature.

Trial drop-outs

The number of drop-outs in the trials reviewed gave cause for concern. The drop-outs were not counted in the trials by Claes and Baert (1993), Colpi et al (1994), Stief et al (1996), Aydin et al (1997), Kho et al (1999) and Mamberti-Dias and Bonierbale-Branchereau (1991). However, in the trials by Claes et al (1995, 1996), Derouet et al (1998), and Van Kampen (1998) a considerable number of patients dropped out. Some subjects failed to perform the required exercise regime, some failed to continue the exercises because of a lack of immediate effect (Claes et al, 1995), whereas others were unwilling to complete the electrical treatment (Derouet et al, 1998). Claes et al (1996a) reported 12 out of 178 (6.7%) men and Claes et al (1995) reported 14 out of 122 (11.4%) who had found it difficult to perform exercises every day. In the trial by Derouet *et al* (1998) a high percentage of men receiving electrical stimulation, 10 out of 48 (20.8%), also dropped out owing to inefficacy or to the stimulation method. This shows the importance of a clear education programme explaining the motivation necessary to complete the expected treatment regime and the need for realistic goals and outcomes.

Outcome measures for erectile dysfunction

Intracavernosal pressure was measured invasively using a pressure transducer (Lavoisier *et al*, 1986; Wespes *et al*, 1990) or non-invasively using a penile cuff (Medasonic) made of non-elastic material filled with water (Lavoisier *et al*, 1988). The penile cuff water pressure correlated with intracavernous pressure ($p < 0.001$).

Mamberti-Dias *et al* (1999) measured the pubo-anal distance from the bulb of the penis to the anterior anal margin to ascertain whether an elongated bulbocavernosus muscle provided a risk factor for erectile dysfunction. Kawanishi *et al* (2000) devised a simple evaluation of the ischiocavernosus muscle by placing a strap round the coronal groove of the penis attached to a spring balance. Maximal contraction power was measured in grams. They found a correlation between the evaluation of maximal contraction power and subnormal pharmacological erection, particularly in patients with veno-occlusive dysfunction.

Most outcomes were defined in three categories: 'cure', 'improved' or 'failure', but Aydin *et al* (1997) defined outcomes in only two categories: 'cure' or 'no response'. 'Cure' was defined as an erection suitable for satisfactory sexual performance with vaginal penetration in all studies. 'Improvement', however, was defined in a number of ways from 'a significant increase of erection quality and performance' (Colpi *et al*, 1994) to 'those who could achieve sexual intercourse but were having some failures' (Aydin *et al*, 1997) and 'partial response for those patients who reported some increase in quality (duration or rigidity) of erections but not sufficient for sexual intercourse' (Claes *et al*, 1995). Only two studies used a method of obtaining independent verification from the partner as to the outcome of treatment (Aydin *et al*, 1997; Kho *et al*, 1999). This method must produce outcomes with greater reliability. Partners should be involved in all aspects of the treatment of erectile dysfunction (Dorey, 2001b).

Van Kampen (2000) added a quality of life evaluation in relation to sexual function in patients at 1, 6, 12 and 15 months after radical prostatectomy. They used a self-administered questionnaire with a seven-point score – excellent, satisfied, content, indifferent, pity, unhappy, unacceptable – in order to gain qualitative outcomes.

Erectile dysfunction questionnaires

The following questionnaires can be used as outcome measures for men with erectile dysfunction (Table 11.2). The International Index of Erectile Function (IIEF) has been developed as a brief and reliable self-administered scale for assessing erectile function (Rosen et al, 1997). It has been validated and is considered to be the gold standard instrument for efficacy assessment in clinical trials. No questionnaires for partners were found.

The erectile dysfunction questionnaires provide varying information concerning the symptoms and extent of erectile dysfunction, as shown in Table 11.3.

Table 11.2 Erectile dysfunction questionnaires

ICSsex	International Continence Society sex questionnaire (Abrams et al, 1997)
PROTOsex	PROstate Trials Office sex instrument (www.proto.org)
Brief SI	Brief Sexual Inventory (O'Leary et al, 1995)
RSSF	Radiumhemmets Scale of Sexual Function (Helgason, 1997)
Veteran	Veterans Affairs Questionnaire (Anonymous, 1993)
IIEF	International Index of Erectile Function (Rosen et al, 1997)
QOL-MED	Quality of Life Male Erectile Dysfunction Questionnaire (Wagner et al, 1996)

Conclusion

There is evidence that the ischiocavernosus and bulbocavernosus muscles increase penile rigidity in the tumescent penis. There is evidence that pelvic floor muscle efficiency is higher in potent than impotent men and that perineal muscle efficiency reduces with age in impotent men. From this literature review, PFMEs using ischiocavernosus and bulbocavernosus muscles seem to have merit as a treatment for erectile dysfunction due to mild or moderate venous leakage and are a realistic alternative to surgery. Men suffering from erectile dysfunction due to other causes may also benefit. Patients also suffering from urinary incontinence and post-micturition dribble (PMD) could combine a simultaneous training programme of PFMEs. There is no strong evidence that electrical stimu-

Table 11.3 Information from erectile dysfunction questionnaires: number of questions in each category

	ICSsex	PROTO	Brief SI	RSSF	Veteran	IIEF	QOL-MED
Rigidity of erections	1	1	4	7		6	1
Psychological aspect							12
Sexual function							1
Orgasmic function			3	7*		1	
Sexual desire			3	2		2	1
Intercourse satisfaction		1		2	1	3	
Ejaculation/volume	1	1		7*		1	
Pain on ejaculation	1	1					
LUTS impact on life	1	1					
Sexual relationship		1				1	10
Overall satisfaction			1			1	
General matters				2			
Urinary difficulty					1		
Activities					1		1
Social activity					1		
General health					1		
Quality of life					1		1
Total number of questions	4	6	11	20	9	15	27

*One question covering two categories.

lation or electro-acupuncture is effective or ineffective. No studies demonstrating preventative conservative treatment were found.

Randomised controlled trials with larger sample numbers are needed to explore the use of pelvic floor exercises as a first line treatment for men with erectile dysfunction. Similar trials are also needed to ascertain the role of pelvic floor exercises as a prevention for erectile dysfunction.

Suggestions for further research

- The number of ischiocavernosus and bulbocavernosus muscle exercises to be performed each day to improve erectile function.
- The number of ischiocavernosus and bulbocavernosus muscle exercises to be performed each day to prevent erectile dysfunction.
- The role of biofeedback in pelvic floor muscle rehabilitation.
- Investigation into whether surface EMG to the pelvic floor is preferable to rectal EMG.

- The effect of electrical stimulation.
- To determine which patients with erectile dysfunction are the best candidates for PFMEs.
- To discover if men suffering from erectile dysfunction also suffer from PMD.
- To determine if the same exercises help erectile dysfunction and PMD.
- To determine if there a role for preventative PFMEs.

Summary

PFMEs using ischiocavernosus and bulbocavernosus muscles seem to have merit as a treatment for erectile dysfunction due to mild or moderate venous leakage. Men suffering from erectile dysfunction due to other causes may also benefit. Patients also suffering from urinary incontinence and PMD could combine a simultaneous training programme of PFMEs.

CHAPTER 12

Setting up a continence service

Integrated continence services

Continence services for a specific population should be organised as integrated continence services (DOH, 2000). The various professionals at different levels may be employed by different bodies but should be integrated into a locally provided continence service. The continence service should comprise the director of continence services, continence nurse specialists, specialist continence physiotherapists, designated medical and surgical specialists, and investigation and treatment facilities.

Each health authority should have access to integrated continence services, managed by a director of continence services who would usually be a continence nurse specialist or specialist continence physiotherapist responsible for:

- overseeing and co-ordinating the development and implementation of common policies, procedures and protocols
- developing and maintaining care pathways to and from primary care and specialist services
- ensuring users and carers are involved in all aspects of the service
- ensuring services are made available to all residents in the area served
- working closely with other services such as social services, education services and psychological services
- ensuring services are made available to all patients in hospital who require them
- co-ordinating educational activities for continence specialists, primary healthcare teams and others involved in the delivery of health and social care

- organising service-wide review, audit and research activities particularly to ensure national targets are met
- promoting awareness of continence (DOH, 2000).

Person specification of director of continence services

The director of continence services should be a continence nurse specialist or a specialist continence physiotherapist who has had considerable experience in the speciality of continence, has good management experience and is able to provide training for members of staff at primary care and secondary care levels.

Qualifications

Physiotherapists may study for the 'Graduate Certificate in Professional Development in Health: Continence' which provides 80 credits at level 3 from the University of East London. This 15 month course includes two study blocks at Leeds and a distance learning package. Students complete a case study or a literature review, a reflective diary and a group presentation. They undertake a required amount of clinical experience, make professional visits and take a practical examination.

Continence courses at level 4 are presently being planned for physiotherapists at Manchester, Middlesex, Glasgow and Oxford Universities.

Nurses may study for the English National Board (ENB) Continence Course 941.

Membership of specialist groups

The specialist continence physiotherapist or continence nurse specialist would be expected to be a member of one or more of the following groups, which provide lectures and courses on continence. All these groups provide benefits to their members such as a directory of specialists, a continence newsletter, shared knowledge from course and conferences, networking, details of current research literature, continence promotions, posters and patient leaflets.

Association for Continence Advice (ACA)

A group for nurses and physiotherapists working in the specialist area of continence.

Association of Chartered Physiotherapists in Women's Health (ACPWH)

A clinical interest group of the Chartered Society of Physiotherapy, which embraces both male and female continence issues.

Chartered Physiotherapists Promoting Continence (CPPC)

A group of physiotherapists who are interested and working in continence therapy, who meet regularly for study days.

International Continence Society (ICS) (UK)

A group which includes doctors, scientists, nurses and physiotherapists from the UK, who are interested in presenting, sharing and hearing the recent research findings.

International Continence Society (ICS)

An international group of doctors, scientists, nurses and physiotherapists who share outcomes from current research.

Continuing professional development

The specialist continence physiotherapist or continence nurse specialist would be expected to attend study days and conferences in order to show evidence of continuing professional development or lifelong learning. The following conferences provide current continence information and evidence on which to base practice:

ACA Conference
ACPWH Conference
CPPC Study Days
Male Continence Study Day
ICS (UK) Conference
ICS Conference

Budget

The following need to be considered when budgeting for a continence service:

- staff salaries
- staff training
- investigative equipment

- biofeedback equipment
- electrical stimulation equipment
- rectal pressure probes, rectal electrodes and surface electrodes
- medical sundries, such as condoms, non-latex gloves and gel
- advertising costs
- patient information leaflet costs
- additional costs for stationery, photocopying, etc.

Business plan

The following considerations should form part of a business plan:

- justification
- quality service
- the internal customers (inpatients, outpatients, home visits, residential homes)
- the external customers (consultants, GPs, carers, and other professionals)
- budget
- audit
- evaluation of services.

Marketing

In order to market the continence service, other professionals and interested parties should be targeted:

- hospital managers
- consultants and GPs
- other nurses, well-man screening programmes, prostate clinics
- other physiotherapists
- the public

The continence service can be advertised by:

- leaflets
- posters
- open days
- lectures to the public
- local paper
- local radio
- local cinema
- local TV

Contacts for specialist groups

Association of Chartered Physiotherapists in Women's Health (ACPWH)
Annual subscription £40
c/o The Chartered Society of Physiotherapy
14 Bedford Row
London WC1R 4ED   Telephone 020 7306 6666

Chartered Physiotherapists Promoting Continence (CPPC)
Annual subscription £15
c/o The Chartered Society of Physiotherapy
14 Bedford Row
London WC1R 4ED   Telephone 020 7306 6666

Association for Continence Advice (ACA)
Annual subscription £30
102a Astra House
Arklow Road
New Cross
London SE14 6EB   Telephone 020 8692 4680
E-mail info@aca.uk.com   Website www.aca.uk.com

Royal College of Nursing Continence Care Forum
20 Cavendish Street
London W1M 0AB   Telephone 020 7409 3333

International Continence Society (ICS) (UK)
Annual subscription £10
www.icsuk.org.uk

International Continence Society (ICS)
Annual subscription £50
ICS Office
Southmead Hospital
Bristol
BS10 5NB   Telephone 0117 950 3510

The membership of professional specialist groups is tax deductable in the UK.

Continence organisations in the UK

The Continence Foundation
    307 Hatton Square
    16 Baldwins Gardens
    London EC1N 7RJ   Telephone 020 7404 6875

Incontinence Information Helpline (Monday–Friday 9a.m.–6p.m.)
    Telephone 0191 213 0050
    Website www.continence-foundation.org.uk

InconTact (National Action on Incontinence)
    United House
    North Road
    London N7 9DP   Telephone 020 7700 7035

Suppliers

Model of the male pelvic floor
    Educational and Scientific Products Ltd
    A2 Dominion Way
    Rustington
    West Sussex BN16 3HQ   Telephone 01903 773340

ANUFORM rectal probe
    NEEN HealthCare
    Old Pharmacy Yard
    Church Street
    Dereham
    Norfolk NR19 1DJ   Telephone 01362 698966

Summary

The continence service should be made up of the director of continence services, continence nurse specialists, specialist continence physiotherapists, designated medical and surgical specialists, and investigation and treatment facilities.

The director may be a continence specialist physiotherapist or a continence nurse specialist with the necessary qualifications and clinical experience.

APPENDIX 1

Assessment forms

Male Subjective Continence Assessment Form

Patient details

Name _____

Address _____

Telephone no. _____

Date of birth/age _____

Occupation _____

Hobbies/activities _____

Source of referral _____

Consultant/GP _____

Problem

Main problem _____

Length of time for main problem _____

Mild   Moderate   Severe

Limitation of activities _____

QOL due to urinary problem _____

Bothersome rating: 0 1 2 3 4 5 6 7 8 9 10

Symptoms

Stress _____

Urgency _____

Urge incontinence _____

Provoking factors _____

Awareness of leakage _____

Frequency_____
Nocturia_____
Nocturnal enuresis_____
Description of flow rate_____
Poor sensation of micturition_____
Hesitation starting to pass urine_____
Difficulty passing urine_____
Weak stream_____
Small voids_____
Terminal dribble_____
Post-void dribble_____
Constant dribble_____
Double void instability (sensation to void again on moving)_____
Does bladder feel empty after voiding_____
Dysuria_____
Haematuria, dark or smoky urine_____
Pain: suprapubic, genital, perineal, testes, penis (mark on body chart)___
Childhood urinary problems_____

Duration of symptoms

Length of time for Symptom 1_____
Length of time for Symptom 2_____
Length of time for Symptom 3_____
Improvement or deterioration to date_____

Severity of symptoms

(visual analogue scale 0–10 for each symptom)
Symptom 1_____0 1 2 3 4 5 6 7 8 9 10
Symptom 2_____0 1 2 3 4 5 6 7 8 9 10
Symptom 3_____0 1 2 3 4 5 6 7 8 9 10

Amount of leakage

Few drops   Spurt   Large leakage
No. of pads per day_____   Damp   Wet   Soaked
Type of appliance_____
ISC_____
In-dwelling catheter_____Size_____Number of days used _____

Frequency of leakage

Daily   >1/week   <1/week   >1/month   <1/month
Time of day leakage occurs_____
Leakage aggravators:
Coughing Sneezing Walking Moving Running water Caffeine Alcohol
Medication   Other:_____

Urine stop test

(not to be used as an exercise)
Stop   Slow down   Unable to stop

Bowel activity

Constipation_____
Straining to defaecate_____
Number of times defaecates per week_____
Stool: Liquid   Soft   Firm
Faecal urgency _____
Faecal incontinence _____
Incontinence of flatus_____
Laxatives_____
Diet_____

Surgical history

TURP____Date_____Outcome_____
Radical prostatectomy_____Date_____Outcome_____
Urethral stricture_____Date_____Outcome_____
Other surgery_____Date_____Outcome_____

Medical history

Family history_____
Prostatitis: Acute_____Chronic_____No. of episodes_____
Cystitis: Acute_____Chronic_____No. of episodes_____
Latex allergy_____
Metal implants_____
Heart problems_____
Smoking_____
Respiratory problems_____

Other problems_____
Anticholinergic medication:
Tolterodine (Detrusitol)_____Oxybutynin (Ditropan)_____
Alpha blockers (relax bladder neck):
Doxazosin mesylate (Cardura)_____
5 alpha reductase inhibitors (reduces size of prostate):
Finasteride (Proscar)_____
Anti-androgen drug treatment_____
Cholinergic agonists (enhance detrusor contractions):
(carbachol, bethanechol)_____
Other medications_____
Effect of medication_____
Side effects of medication_____
Radiotherapy_____
Neurological problems:
Diabetes MS Parkinson's Other_____
Lumbar or cervical spine problems with neurological deficit_____

Previous treatment

Previous physiotherapy and outcome_____

Body mass index

Height_____metres
Weight_____kilograms
BMI (weight in kilograms divided by height in metres squared: >30 = obese)

Sexual problems

Difficulty gaining erection_____
Difficulty maintaining erection_____
Premature ejaculation_____

Functional factors

Position used for urination_____
Mobility and dexterity_____
Environmental factors_____
Cognitive/mental abilities _____
Psychological state_____
Patient support system_____

Motivation

Ability to incorporate therapy into lifestyle_____

Investigations

Urinalysis of MSU (essential)_____
Prostate specific antigen (men>50 and <75) (of interest)_____
Uroflow (essential if physio is 1st contact)_____
Post void residual (essential if physio is 1st contact)_____
Ultrasound scan (of interest)_____
Urodynamics including post-void residual and uroflow (helpful)_____
Flexible cystoscopy for diagnosis of stricture and tumours (helpful)_____
Pad test (preferably 24 hours) (useful to assess treatment effects)_____

Frequency/volume chart

(home and work days; ideally 7 days)
Frequency of voiding_____
Maximum voided volume_____
Minimum voided volume_____
Amount of fluid intake_____
Amount of caffeine intake_____
Amount of alcohol intake_____
Amount of urinary output_____
Time of going to bed_____
Amount voided at night (polyuria > 33 % of 24 hour volume)_____
Frequency of leakage_____
Number of pads per day_____

Male Objective Continence Assessment Form

Informed consent:

Abdominal palpation

Distended abdomen_____
Abdominal pain_____

Perineal and genital examination
(in crook lying)
Congenital abnormality_____

Skin condition (penis, perineum and rectal area)_____
Evidence of infection_____
Ability to tighten anus_____
Ability to contract PFMs and perform penile dip and scrotal lift_____
Leakage on coughing_____
Ability to prevent leakage on coughing_____

Dermatomes
S2 lateral buttocks and thigh, posterior calf and plantar heel_____
S3 upper two-thirds of medial thigh_____
S4 penis and perineal area_____

Myotomes
External anal sphincter S2 and S3_____
Levator ani, ischiococcygeus and bulbocavernosus and bladder S2–4___

Reflexes
Bulbocavernosus reflex_____
(gentle pressure on the glans penis during a DRE elicits anal sphincter contraction unless neurological impairment)

Digital rectal examination

Anterior

O

Posterior

Sensation of right side of pelvic floor_____
Sensation of left side of pelvic floor_____
Integrity of right side of anal sphincter_____
Integrity of left side of anal sphincter_____
Action of puborectalis_____
Prostate tested in side lying after training (refer if craggy or hard nodule)_
Pelvic floor strength   0 1 2 3 4 5
Pelvic floor endurance_____
Number of repetitions_____
Ability to perform fast contraction_____

Problems

1
2
3
4

Patient identified goals of treatment

1
2
3
4

Treatment

1
2
3
4

Advice

1
2
3
4

Plan

1
2
3
4

Questions for next time

1
2
3
4

Name of physiotherapist_____

Signature_____

Date _____

Patient information leaflets

Can you hold your beer?

Beer, like most alcoholic drinks, causes you to pass urine more frequently – in technical terms, it is a diuretic. Greater input causes greater output. The number of pints passed from the bladder reflects the number of pints drunk. So drinking late in the evening is one reason for having to get up at night to go to the bathroom. Another reason may be the diuretic effect of some prescribed drugs or over-the-counter medicines such as decongestants. It's also partly to do with your age. As people get older, their kidneys (where the urine is made) work better at night and produce more urine then.

Effect of caffeine

Products containing caffeine can also affect the way your bladder behaves, by making the bladder muscle more active. Too much caffeine can make you feel a strong urge to pass urine.

Coffee, tea, cocoa, chocolate and cola drinks all contain caffeine. Because we are a nation of tea and coffee drinkers, we do not stop to question whether these beverages are good for our health. Our 'Never mind, have a cup of tea', 'Stay awake with coffee' society has a lot to answer for. Too much caffeine can also cause headaches, nausea, irritability, tremor and palpitations.

So, to help prevent bladder problems, **avoid:**
coffee
tea
chocolate
cocoa
cola

and remember that some medicines can also cause problems:
decongestant medicines
allergy medicines.

So what are we to drink?

Water is the purest and best drink and the optimum thirst quencher. Decaffeinated coffee and tea are now widely available in most supermarkets. But a word of warning – if you suddenly cut out caffeine from your diet you may experience withdrawal symptoms of headaches or sleepiness. So reduce your caffeine levels gradually. Cutting out caffeine will help reduce unwanted bladder contractions. If you are setting out on a long car journey, choose a caffeine-free drink before you leave.

It is important not to limit your fluid intake. Drinking too little fluid leads to concentrated urine and the risk of urinary infections. Also, in the long run, the bladder will lose its elasticity and stretchiness. Keep up your fluid level, especially during and after strenuous exercise. If your urine is darker in colour in a hot climate, while you are travelling, or after exercise, you need to drink more water.

Some **drinks without caffeine** are:
water
decaffeinated coffee
decaffeinated tea
decaffeinated cola
herb tea
milk
apple juice
cranberry juice
blackcurrant juice

Can you hold on until you get there?

For some men the urge to pass urine is so violent that they leak before they reach the toilet. In severe cases these violent contractions can lead to bedwetting. What can be done to help?

- Reducing your intake of caffeine and alcohol will help to prevent unwanted bladder contractions and the urge to pass urine.
- Strong pelvic floor muscles will help to prevent the urine escaping.
- Always ensure the bladder is fully emptied before you go to bed.

The secret is having strong pelvic floor muscles

As with all the muscles in the body, weakness comes from lack of exercise. It isn't only women who suffer from weak pelvic floor muscles. Today's 'use it or lose it' men know that regular exercise promotes healthy function. Pelvic floor exercises can help by producing better muscle tone in the pelvic floor and therefore better control of urination. These exercises can also be used in the treatment of premature ejaculation and some forms of erectile dysfunction.

Where is the pelvic floor?

Your pelvic floor is the part of you that you would sit on if you were riding a horse. It is a sheet of muscle like a hammock that extends from your tail bone to your pubic bone at the front. It supports the contents of your abdomen, allows the passage of urine and faeces and has a function in sexual activity.

Do you know how to exercise your pelvic floor?

A Chartered Physiotherapist who specialises in men's health will be able to help you.

- If you stand up and tighten your back passage to prevent wind from escaping, you are tightening your pelvic floor at the back.
- If you tighten up at the front to prevent urine escaping, you are tightening your pelvic floor at the front.

Try tightening at the front and holding for 3 seconds (or for the number of seconds your physiotherapist has assessed that you can manage) as hard as you can. By tightening as strongly as you can, you can build up your muscle power. Make sure you are not holding your breath or pulling your tummy in or clenching your buttocks. Repeat this exercise 3 times. Each time you tighten, you will find the base of your penis moves towards your abdomen and your scrotum lifts so you will know you are doing a correct lifting and tightening technique. Now try sitting down and repeating the same exercise as strongly as you can.

You may like to try tightening when you are lying down. Lie on your back and bend your knees up, keeping your feet on the bed, and tighten up your pelvic floor in this position. Each tightening should be as strong as possible, held for 3 seconds and gradually released.

As you get stronger (or when your physiotherapist has indicated following an assessment) you may like to increase your holding time to 4 seconds and, as you improve, up to 10 seconds. You might like to try a quick contraction by tightening fast and then letting go, or try a fast contraction followed by holding for 3 or more seconds. This tightening enables you to recruit these muscles speedily, when you need to give added control.

Secret exercises

Exercises may be performed at any time without anyone noticing. You may like to perform 3 slow contractions lying down, 3 contractions sitting up and 3 contractions while standing, twice a day. It is a good idea to do your exercises in a variety of positions. You could exercise your pelvic floor muscles at the traffic lights or when you are waiting for a telephone call. Now try lifting your pelvic floor 50% while you are standing. If you have control of these muscles, you can tighten while you are walking. Gradually you will become sufficiently expert to tighten your pelvic floor while you are getting out of a chair, or while you are coughing, sneezing or lifting.

Many men who have leakage of urine, for example after a prostate operation, find that they can help themselves to regain control by tightening the pelvic floor muscles before they undertake activities. Men who comply with their exercise regime may recover at a much faster rate than those who forget to practise. After recovery from surgery a maintenance exercise programme is recommended for life.

Why is there sometimes a leakage after a prostate operation?

The prostate gland is situated below the neck of the bladder and in front of the rectum (the lower part of the bowel). Its function is to produce fluid which allows sperm to move and stay alive.

The prostate enlarges with age, and may partly block the urethra (the pipe from the bladder) causing problems such as

- a weak, slow or intermittent stream of urine
- difficulty in initiating urination
- excessive straining to urinate
- the feeling of incomplete emptying.

In severe cases, as the prostate gradually enlarges with age it can block the urethra altogether and stop the passage of urine. If a large amount of urine is being retained in the bladder, a man may need an operation called prostatectomy to relieve the blockage. In this operation the sphincter or ring of muscle around the neck of the bladder is removed, along with the part of the enlarged prostate that is blocking the urethra. If the pelvic floor muscles are weak, there may be some leakage of urine after the operation.

Will physiotherapy help after a prostate operation?

Physiotherapy can help to strengthen the pelvic floor muscles.

- Preventative pelvic floor muscle exercises before the operation may help to avoid leakage afterwards.
- The physiotherapist may use biofeedback to let you see how well you are progressing.
- The pelvic floor muscles may be stimulated by electrotherapy, to make the muscles contract. This treatment is safe and does not hurt but you may feel a tingling sensation.

Do you dribble after urinating?

If you leak after you have passed urine, try tightening your pelvic floor muscles after you have finished urinating. Something else that might help is massaging the remaining urine out from the 'kink' in the urethra (the pipe carrying urine from the bladder).

- After urinating, tighten your pelvic floor muscles to 'squeeze out'.
- Then place one hand on your pelvic floor behind your scrotum, and massage gently but firmly upwards and forwards to push the urine out of the bend in the urethra.
- Shaking your penis will help to get rid of the last few drops.

Can you cut down your trips to the bathroom?

Normally men pass urine 6 to 8 times in 24 hours, but this may vary slightly for a variety of reasons such as the size of your bladder and the amount you drink. However, if you are passing urine 10 or more times in 24 hours, you may like to try cutting down your trips to the bathroom.

- Tightening your pelvic floor muscles may help; so does sitting down on a firm chair, or just standing still.

- Many men find that if they stay calm the urge to pass urine will disappear and they can resume their normal activities without needing to void urine.
- If you can cut down the number of visits to the bathroom during the day, you may find that the night-time visits are often reduced too.

Do you suffer from constipation?

Constipation makes bladder symptoms worse, because the pressure from a distended bowel pushes on the bladder. This causes urgency, frequency and sometimes incomplete emptying of the bladder.

- Try to avoid constipation by drinking enough liquids, walking regularly, and eating plenty of fresh vegetables and fibre (roughage).
- Straining to pass a motion weakens the pelvic floor muscles, and the impacted stool may irritate the bladder.
- Avoid laxatives and enemas, because if you use them regularly the normal function of the bowel will decrease.
- You may wish to discuss your diet with a dietician.

Now can you hold your beer?

So, to sum up, here's how you can look after your health and still be able to hold your beer:
- drink alcohol in moderation
- cut out caffeine
- drink at least 6–8 normal sized cups a day of fluid (without alcohol or caffeine)
- eat healthily
- avoid constipation
- walk regularly
- secretly exercise your pelvic floor muscles.

Men in control: How physiotherapy can help your pelvic floor

Men can suffer from a variety of problems with passing urine, especially as they get older. Sometimes the only sign that changes are happening may be a desire to pass urine more often, or a need to pass water urgently, or an increased number of visits to the bathroom at night. Sometimes leakage of urine may occur.

Often these problems are caused by changes in the prostate gland. The prostate is situated below the neck of the bladder and in front of the rectum (the lower part of the bowel). Its function is to produce fluid which allows sperm to move and stay alive.

It is normal for the prostate to enlarge with age. However, because it is located so close to the bladder this may eventually cause a blockage of the urethra (the pipe carrying urine from the bladder), causing various problems:

- a weak, slow or intermittent stream of urine
- difficulty in starting to urinate
- excessive straining to urinate
- the feeling of incomplete emptying.

If the obstruction is severe, or if a large amount of urine is being retained, a man may need an operation called a prostatectomy to relieve the blockage. In this operation the sphincter or ring of muscle around the neck of the bladder is removed, along with the part of the enlarged prostate which blocks the urethra. If the pelvic floor muscles are weak, there may be some leakage of urine after the operation.

This leaflet shows you ways of preventing urine leakage by strengthening your pelvic floor muscles. It also suggests ways of coping with some of the other symptoms already mentioned.

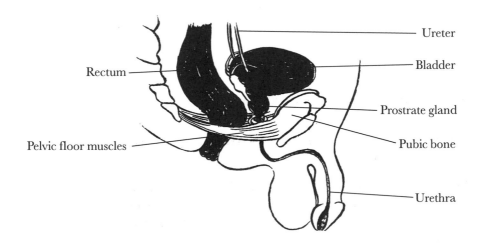

Diagram of the prostate.

Pelvic floor muscle exercises

Your pelvic floor is the part of you that you would sit on if you were riding a horse. It is a sheet of muscle that extends from your tail bone to your pubic bone at the front, like a hammock.

If you stand up and tighten your back passage to prevent wind from escaping you are tightening your pelvic floor at the back.

If you stand up and tighten up at the front to prevent passing water you are tightening your pelvic floor at the front.

Try tightening at the front and holding for 3 seconds (or for the number of seconds your physiotherapist has assessed that you can manage) as hard as you can. By tightening as strongly as you can, you can build up your muscle power. Make sure you are not holding your breath or pulling your tummy in or clenching your buttocks. Repeat this exercise 3 times. Each time you tighten, you will find the base of your penis moves towards your abdomen and your scrotum lifts so you will know you are doing a correct lifting and tightening technique. Now try sitting down and repeating the same exercise as strongly as you can.

You may like to try tightening when you are lying down. Lie on your back and bend your knees up, keeping your feet on the bed, and tighten up your pelvic floor in this position. Each tightening should be as strong as possible, held for 3 seconds and gradually released.

As you get stronger (or when your physiotherapist has indicated following an assessment) you may like to increase your holding time to 4 seconds and, as you improve, up to 10 seconds. You might like to try a quick contraction by tightening fast and then letting go, or try a fast contraction followed by holding for 3 or more seconds. This tightening enables you to recruit these muscles speedily, when you need to give added control.

Home exercises

You can do these exercises at any time without anyone noticing. You may like to perform 3 slow contractions lying down, 3 contractions sitting up and 3 contractions while standing, twice a day. It is a good idea to do your exercises in a variety of positions. Now try lifting your pelvic floor 50% while you are standing. If you have control of these muscles, you can tighten them while you are walking.

Gradually you will become expert enough to tighten your muscles firmly just before coughing, sneezing or lifting. Many men find that by tightening before doing things like this, they can help themselves to regain control.

Men who are committed to their exercise regime, and comply with it, recover from a prostate operation much faster than those who forget to practise. After recovery a maintenance exercise programme is recommended for life.

Some recent research has shown that pelvic floor exercises have helped in the treatment of some types of erectile dysfunction and also as a treatment for premature ejaculation.

Electrotherapy

The pelvic floor muscles may be stimulated by electrotherapy to make the muscles contract. This treatment is safe and does not hurt but you may feel a tingling sensation. Electrotherapy may also help to reduce the urge to urinate.

Standing to urinate

Standing up to urinate is a more functional position than sitting. Your muscles will work better in a standing position.

Dribbling after urinating

If you leak after you have passed urine, try tightening your pelvic floor muscles after you have finished urinating. Something else that might help is massaging the remaining urine out from the 'kink' in the urethra (the pipe carrying urine from the bladder).

- After urinating, tighten your pelvic floor muscles and 'squeeze out'.
- Then place one hand on your pelvic floor behind your scrotum, and massage gently but firmly upwards and forwards to push the urine out of the bend in the urethra.
- Shaking your penis will help to get rid of the last few drops.

Getting up at night to pass urine

There are many reasons why men have to get up at night to visit the bathroom.

- Perhaps you have drunk too much fluid during the day or before going to bed.
- Perhaps you have had too many drinks containing caffeine.
- Perhaps you have drunk too much alcohol

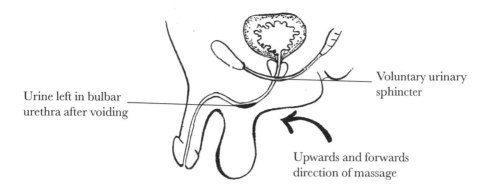

Diagram of bulbar massage.

- Some drugs (prescribed or over-the-counter) make you pass more urine.
- As you age, the kidneys function better at night and this increases the production of urine.

Frequency/volume chart

Your physiotherapist may give you a chart called a frequency/volume chart to fill in, to help monitor your bladder activity. From this, the physiotherapist can find out the size of your bladder, the amount of urine you pass in 24 hours, the amount you drink in 24 hours, the type of fluids you drink and how often you go to the bathroom. The physiotherapist will then be able to give you the correct advice and help your specific problem.

Can you cut down your trips to the bathroom?

Normally men pass urine 6 to 8 times in 24 hours, but this may vary slightly for a variety of reasons such as the size of your bladder and the amount you drink. However, if you are passing urine 10 or more times in 24 hours, you may like to try cutting down your trips to the bathroom.

- Tightening your pelvic floor muscles may help; so does sitting down on a firm chair, or just standing still.
- Many men find that if they stay calm the urge to pass urine will disappear and they can resume their normal activities without needing to void urine.

- If you can cut down the number of visits to the bathroom during the day, you may find that the night-time visits are often reduced too.

Caffeine products

Caffeine is contained in products such as coffee, tea, cocoa, chocolate and cola. Drinking strong coffee regularly can cause havoc to the lining of the bladder, strong urges to urinate, and unwanted contractions of the bladder associated with a large leakage of urine. In severe cases it can even cause bedwetting.

Many men find that these urges will disappear if they change to drinking decaffeinated products. But change your drinking habits gradually. It is not a good idea to stop caffeine products suddenly, because you may get withdrawal symptoms such as headaches or sleepiness.

Drinking water is best!

Constipation

Try to avoid constipation, because straining weakens the pelvic floor muscles and hard stool retained in the bowel may irritate the bladder. You may wish to discuss your diet with a dietician.

Pelvic floor muscle exercises for men

Standing up

Stand with your feet apart and tighten your pelvic floor muscles as if you were trying to stop the flow of urine. If you look in a mirror, you should be able to see the base of your penis move nearer to your abdomen and your testicles rise.

- Hold the contraction as strongly as you can.
- Try to avoid pulling in your abdomen or tensing your buttocks.
- Perform 3 maximal contractions in the **morning**, holding for ___ seconds.
- Perform 3 maximal contractions in the **evening**, holding for ___ seconds.

Sitting down

Sit on a chair with your knees apart and tighten your pelvic floor muscles as if you were lifting your pelvic floor off a drawing pin.

- Hold the contraction as strongly as you can.
- Try to avoid pulling in your abdomen or tensing your buttocks.
- Perform 3 maximal contractions in the **morning**, holding for ___ seconds.
- Perform 3 maximal contractions in the **evening**, holding for ___ seconds.

Lying down

Lie on your back with your knees bent and your knees apart. Tighten your pelvic floor and hold the contraction as strongly as you can.

- Try to avoid pulling in your abdomen or tensing your buttocks.
- Perform 3 maximal contractions in the **morning**, holding for ___ seconds.
- Perform 3 maximal contractions in the **evening**, holding for ___ seconds.

While walking

Try lifting your pelvic floor up 50% when walking.

After urinating

After you have passed urine, try tightening your pelvic floor muscles **strongly** to avoid the embarrassing after-dribble.

During sexual activity

Try tightening your pelvic floor muscles rhythmically to achieve and maintain penile rigidity during sexual activity. **Slow** thrusting movements generate higher pressures inside the penis.

To delay ejaculation

Try tightening your pelvic floor muscles to delay premature ejaculation.

'The knack'

Try tightening just before and during activities which increase your abdominal pressure such as coughing, sneezing, lifting and getting out of a chair.

Lifestyle changes for men with erectile dysfunction

There are a number of ways in which you can change your lifestyle to become generally fitter. These changes may help to improve your penile erections.

Alcohol

Drinking too much alcohol can lead to erectile difficulties. Try to reduce your daily intake to 2 units of alcohol a day or less (1 pint of beer or 2 whiskies or 2 glasses of wine).

	0	2	4	6	8	10 units a day
Record						

Smoking

Smoking is bad for the blood circulation. This may produce erectile difficulties. This may be the excuse you need to give up smoking. There are leaflets and support groups which may help you.

NHS Smoking Helpline 0800 169 0169

	0	10	20	30	40	50 a day
Record						

General fitness

Being unfit can put a strain on the heart and the blood pressure, and this can cause erectile difficulties. You can gradually increase your fitness by walking every day and then building up your fitness level by swimming, by sport or by exercising in a gym at least twice a week.

	Walking	Exercise 1 × week	Exercise 2 × week	Daily exercise
Record				

Weight

Being seriously overweight can put a strain on the heart and lead to high blood pressure, and this in turn can affect penile erection. You may find it helpful to join a weight reduction group.

Correct weight 1 stone over 2 stone over 3 stone over 4 stone over
Record   _____

Cycling

Cycling can affect the blood circulation to the pelvic floor and the penis. The saddle pressure from prolonged cycling may also damage the nerves to the penis. Try a change of saddle, or taking breaks during your cycle ride, or lifting yourself up from the saddle from time to time.

     Not cycling   5 miles   10 miles   20 miles   40 miles
Record   _____

Glossary and abbreviations

ACA Association for Continence Advice
ACPWH Association of Chartered Physiotherapists in Women's Health
ANV actual number of nightly voids
AUA American Urologic Association
AVP arginine vasopressin
PBDIR perineobulbar detrusor inhibitory reflex
BCM bulbocavernosus muscle (also called bulbospongiosus muscle)
BFB biofeedback (monitors muscle activity to encourage greater muscular effort)
BMI body mass index (over 30 is obese)
BOO bladder outlet obstruction
BPE benign prostatic enlargement
BPH benign prostatic hyperplasia
Brief SI Brief Sexual Inventory
cardiac arrhythmia irregular heartbeat
cmH2O centimetres of water
CPPC Chartered Physiotherapists Promoting Continence
Credé's manoeuvre leaning forward with pressure on the abdomen while straining to void
cyclopegia blurred vision
cystometry tests relationship between volume and pressure in bladder during filling and voiding
cystourethroscopy endoscopic investigation of the bladder & urethra
DAN-PSS-1 Danish Prostatic Symptom Score
detrusor/sphincter dyssynergia spasm of the internal urethral sphincter while the bladder is contracting
DDFR detrusodetrusor facilitative reflex

DDV deep dorsal vein incision (penile venous incision or ligation or embolisation) reduces the number of channels for venous outflow from the penis and therefore increases venous resistance

DOB date of birth

DRE digital rectal examination

DSIR detrusosphincteric inhibitory reflex

DUIR detrusourethral inhibitory reflex

dysuria pain on passing urine

ED erectile dysfunction (the inability to achieve or maintain an erection sufficient for satisfactory performance)

EMG electromyogram (the monitoring of muscle activity by electronic means using skin electrodes, or a rectal electrode or from a needle electrode)

ENB English National Board

epistaxis nose bleed

ES electrical stimulation (of muscle to achieve a muscle contraction)

FBC functional bladder capacity

flatus wind from the back passage

F/V chart frequency/volume chart

GP general practitioner

gynaecomastia development of breasts in a man

Hz Hertz (unit of frequency of electrical current)

iatrogenic trauma caused by surgery or medication

ICM ischiocavernosus muscle

ICP intracavernous pressure (pressure within the cavernous corpora of the penis)

ICS International Continence Society

ICSsex International Continence Society sex questionnaire

idiopathic no known cause

IIEF International Index of Erectile Function

I-PSS International Prostate Symptom Score

ISC intermittent self-catheterisation

ISIR International Society of Impotence Research

ISMR index of subjective mean rigidity (measure of penile rigidity by the patient)

isometric contraction static contraction of muscle with same length

isotonic contraction dynamic contraction of muscle with same tone

libido sexual urge

IVP Intravenous pyelogram

KUB Xray of kidneys, ureter and bladder

LUTS lower urinary tract symptoms
mg milligram
ml millilitre
MMAP Maine Medical Assessment Program
mmHg millimetres of mercury
ms milliseconds
MS multiple sclerosis
MSU mid-stream urine
μV microvolt
natriuresis excretion of sodium ions
NBCI nocturnal bladder capacity index
ng/ml nanograms/millilitre
NI nocturia index
NIH National Institutes of Health
NPI nocturnal polyuria index
NUV nocturnal urine volume
orchidectomy surgical removal of the testis
PBDFR perineobulbar detrusor facilitative reflex
PDIR perineodetrusor inhibitory reflex
PFMs pelvic floor muscles
PFMEs pelvic floor muscle exercises (contractions of all the pelvic floor muscles)
pH percentage hydrogen
PMD post-micturition dribble
PNV predicted number of nightly voids
PPFR perineopudendal facilitative reflex
PROTOsex PROstate Trials Office sex instrument
PSA prostate specific antigen
PVD post-void dribble
Q_{max} maximum urinary flow rate
QOL quality of life
QOL-MED Quality of Life Male Erectile Dysfunction Questionnaire
RCT randomised controlled trial
RSSF Radiumhemmets Scale of Sexual Function
SDIR sympathetic detrusor inhibiting reflex
SSCR sympathetic sphincter-constrictor reflex
tachycardia increased heartbeat
TURP transurethral resection of prostate
UDFR urethrodetrusor facilitative reflex

urodynamics study of pressure, volume and flow relationships in the lower urinary tract

USGR urethrosphincteric guarding reflex

USIR urethrosphincteric inhibitory reflex

Valsalva manoeuvre bearing down as if defaecating

Veteran Veterans Affairs Questionnaire

VL venous leakage (of blood from the veins in the penis compromising penile rigidity)

WHO World Health Organisation

xanthines natural diuretics such as caffeine and theobromine

References

Abrams P (1994) New words for old: lower urinary tract symptoms for 'prostatism'. British Medical Journal 308: 929–930.

Abrams P (1995) Managing lower urinary tract symptoms in older men. British Medical Journal 310: 1113–1117.

Abrams P, Donovan JL, de la Rosette JJMCM, Scafer W and the ICS BPH Study Group (1997) International Continence Society 'Benign Prostatic Hyperplasia' Study: background, aims and methodology. Neurourology and Urodynamics 16: 79–91.

Abrams P, Freeman R, Anderström C, Mattiasson A (1998a) Tolterodine, a new antimuscarinic agent: as effective but better tolerated than oxybutynin in patients with an over active bladder. British Journal of Urology 81: 801–810.

Abrams PA, Blaivas JG, Stanton SL, Andersen JT (1998b) Standardization of the lower urinary tract function. Neurourology and Urodynamics 7: 403.

ACA (2000) Survey of Patients National Care Audit. London: Association for Continence Advice.

Addison R (1997) Cranberry juice: the story so far. Journal of the Association of Chartered Physiotherapists in Women's Health 80: 21–22.

Albaugh J, Lewis JH (1999) Insights into the management of erectile dysfunction: Part I. Urologic Nursing 19(4): 241–247.

Amarenco G, Lanoe Y, Perrigot M, Goudal H (1987) Un nouveau syndrome canalaire: la compression du nerf honteux interne dans le canal d'Alcock ou paralysie périnéale du cycliste. Presses Médicales 16: 399.

Andersen KV, Bovim G (1997) Impotence and nerve entrapment in long distance amateur cyclists. Acta Neurologica Scandinavica 95(4): 233–240.

Andrew J, Nathan PW, Spanos NC (1964) Cerebral cortex and micturition. Proceedings of the Royal Society of Medicine 58: 533.

Anonymous (1993) A comparison of quality of life with patient reported symptoms and objective findings of men with benign prostatic hyperplasia. The Department of Veterans Affairs Cooperative Study of transurethral resection for benign prostatic hyperplasia. Journal of Urology 150: 1696–1700.

Ashton-Miller JA, DeLancey JOL (1996) The knack: use of precisely-timed pelvic muscle contraction can reduce leakage in SUI. Neurourology and Urodynamics 15(4): 392–393.

Avorn J, Monane M, Gurwitz JH et al (1994) Reduction of bacteriuria and pyuria after ingestion of cranberry juice. JAMA 271: 751–754.

Aydin S, Ercan M, Çaskurlu T *et al* (1997) Acupuncture and hypnotic suggestions in the treatment of non-organic male sexual dysfunction. Scandinavian Journal of Urology and Nephrology 31: 271-274.

Aytac IA, McKinlay JB, Krane RJ (1999) The likely worldwide increase in erectile dysfunction between 1995 and 2025 and some possible policy consequences. British Journal of Urology International 84: 50–56.

Bales GT, Gerber GS, Minor TX *et al* (2000) Effect of preoperative biofeedback/pelvic floor training on continence in men undergoing radical prostatectomy. Adult Urology 56(4): 627–630.

Ballard DJ (1997) Treatment of erectile dysfunction: can pelvic muscle exercises improve sexual function? Journal of Wound Ostomy and Continence Nurses 24: 255-264.

Barrett DM, Wein AJ (1991) Voiding dysfunction: diagnosis, classification and management. In: Gillenwater JY, Grayhack JT, Howards SS, Duckett JW (eds) Adult Pediatric Urology, 2nd edn. Chicago: Mosby-YearBook.

Barry MJ, Fowler FJ, O'Leary MP *et al* (1992) The American Urological Association Symptom Index for Benign Prostatic Hyperplasia. Journal of Urology 148: 1549–1557.

Barry MJ, Fowler FJ, O'Leary MP *et al* (1995) Measuring disease-specific health status in men with benign prostatic hyperplasia. Medical Care 33: AS145–AS155.

Beachy EH (1981) Bacterial adherence; adhesion receptor inter-actions mediating the attachment of bacteria to mucosal surfaces. Journal of Infectious Diseases 143: 325–345.

Benet AE, Melman A (1995) The epidemiology of erectile dysfunction. Urologic Clinics of North America 22: 699–709.

Bennett JK, Foote JE, Green BG, Killorin EW, Martin SH (1997) Effectiveness of biofeedback/electrostimulation in treatment of post-prostatectomy urinary incontinence (abstract). Urodynamics Society meeting, April 1997, New Orleans.

Bensignor MF, Labat JJ, Robert R, Ducrot P (1996) Diagnostic and therapeutic pudendal nerve blocks for patients with perineal non-malignant pain (abstract). 8th World Congress on Pain, 1996, p. 56.

Benton LA, Baker LL, Bowman BR, Waters RL (1981) Functional stimulation: A practical clinical guide. Rancho Los Amigos Rehabilitation Engineering Centre, California, pp. 1-78.

Berger Y (1995) Urodynamic studies. In: Fitzpatrick JM, Krane RJ (eds) The Bladder. London: Churchill Livingstone, pp. 119–128.

Berghmans LCM, Hendriks HJM, Bø K, Hay-Smith EJ, de Bie RA and van Waalwijk van Doorn ESC (1998) Conservative treatment of stress urinary incontinence in women: a systematic review of randomized clinical trials. British Journal of Urology 82: 181–191.

Bernstein IT (1997) The pelvic floor muscles: muscle thickness in healthy and urinary-incontinent women measured by perineal ultrasonography with reference to the effect of pelvic floor training. Estrogen receptor studies. Neurourology and Urodynamics 16: 237–275.

Blaivas JG, Appell RA, Fanti JA *et al* (1997) Definition and classification of urinary incontinence: Recommendations of the Urodynamic Society. Neurourology and Urodynamics 16: 149–151.

Bø K (1994) Techniques. In: Shussler B, Laycock J, Norton P, Stanton S (eds) Pelvic Floor Re-education. Principle and Practice. London: Springer-Verlag, pp. 134–139.

Bø K (1995) Pelvic floor muscle exercise for the treatment of stress urinary incontinence: an exercise physiology perspective. International Urogynecology Journal 6: 282–291.

Bodel PT, Cotran R, Kass EH (1959) Cranberry juice and antibacterial action of hippuric acid. Journal of Laboratory and Clinical Medicine 54(6): 881–888.

Bolognese JA, Kozloff RC, Kumitz SC et al (1992) Validation of a symptoms questionnaire for benign prostatic hyperplasia. Prostate 21: 247–254.

Boolell M, Geri-attee S, Gingell JC et al (1996) Sildenafil, a novel effective oral therapy for male erectile dysfunction. British Journal of Urology 78: 257–261.

Bortolotti A, Parazzini F, Colli E, Landoni M (1997) The epidemiology of erectile dysfunction and its risk factors. International Journal of Andrology 20(6): 323–334.

Boyarsky S, Jones G, Paulson DF, Prout GR (1977) A new look at bladder neck obstruction by the Food and Drug Administration regulators: guidelines for investigation of benign prostatic hypertrophy. Transactions of the American Association of Genito-Urinary Surgery 68: 29–32.

Branch LG, Walker LA, Wetle TT, DuBeau CE, Resnick NM (1994) Urinary incontinence knowledge among community-dwelling people 65 years of age and older. Journal of the American Geriatric Society 42(12): 1257–1262.

Britton JP, Dowell AC, Whelan P (1990) Prevalence of urinary symptoms in men aged over 60. British Journal of Urology 66: 175–176.

Brock GB, Lue TF (1993) Drug-induced male sexual dysfunction: an update. Drug Safety 8(6): 414–426.

Brocklehurst JC (1993) Urinary incontinence in the community – analysis of a MORI poll. British Medical Journal 306: 832–834.

Bump RC, Hurt WG, Fantl JA, Wyman JA (1991) Assessment of Kegel pelvic muscle exercise performance after brief verbal instruction. American Journal of Obstetrics and Gynecology 165: 322–329.

Burgio KL, Stutzman RE, Engel BT (1989) Behavioral training for post-prostatectomy urinary incontinence. Journal of Urology 141: 303–306.

Butler RN, Lewis MI, Hoffman E, Whitehead ED (1994) Love and sex after 60: how to evaluate and treat the impotent older man. A round table discussion: Part 2. Geriatrics 2(49): 27–32.

Caldamone AA (1994) Embryology. In: Sant GR (ed) Pathophysiologic Principles of Urology. Oxford: Blackwell Scientific, pp. 1–29.

Castleden CM, Duffin HM, Gulati RS (1986) Double blind study of imipramine and placebo for incontinence due to bladder instability. Age and Ageing 15: 299–303.

Chamberlain J, Melia J, Moss S, Brown J (1997) Report prepared for the health technology assessment panel of the NHS executive on the diagnosis, management, treatment and costs of prostate cancer in England and Wales. British Journal of Urology 79(3): 1–32.

Chang PL, Tsai LH, Huang ST et al (1998) The early effect of pelvic floor muscle exercise after transurethral prostatectomy. Journal of Urology 160(2): 402–405.

Chapple CR, Parkhouse H, Gardner G, Milroy EJG (1990) Double-blind, placebo controlled cross over study of flavoxate in the treatment of idiopathic detrusor instability. British Journal of Urology 66: 491–494.

Chaudry AA, Booth CM, Holmes A, Al-Dabbagh MA (1997) Are urodynamics essential for the management of 'prostatism'? Two patient group studies. British Journal of Urology 79 (Suppl 4): 18.

Christensen H, Huglsang-Frederiksen A (1998) Quantitative surface EMG during sustained and intermittent submaximal contractions. Electroencephalography and Clinical Neurophysiology 70(3): 239–247.

Chung WS, Sohn JH, Park YY (1999) Is obesity an underlying factor in erectile dysfunction? European Urology 36(1): 68–70.

Chute CG, Panser LA, Girman CJ et al (1993) The prevalence of prostatism: a population-based survey of urinary symptoms. Journal of Urology 150: 85–89.

Claes H, Baert L (1993) Pelvic floor exercise versus surgery in the treatment of impotence. British Journal of Urology 71: 52–57.

Claes H, van Hove J, van de Voorde W *et al* (1993) Pelvi-perineal rehabilitation for dysfunctioning erections. A clinical and anatomo-physiologic study. International Journal of Impotence Research 5(1): 13–26.

Claes H, Kampen M Van, Lysens R, Baert L (1995) Pelvic floor exercises in the treatment of impotence. European Journal of Physical Medicine and Rehabilitation 5. 135–140.

Claes HIM, Vandenbroucke HB, Baert LV (1996a) Pelvic floor exercise in the treatment of impotence. Journal of Urology Supplement 157(4): 786.

Claes H, Bijnens B, Baert L (1996b) The hemodynamic influence of the ischiocavernosus muscles on erectile function. Journal of Urology 156: 986–990.

Cliff AM, McDonagh RP, Speakman MJ *et al* (1997) Further validation of the I-PSS questionnaire. British Journal of Urology 79 (Suppl 4): 12 (poster).

Cockett AT, Aso Y, Denis LJ, Khoury S (1991) Recommendations of the International Consensus Committee. Program Urology 1: 957–972.

Colpi GM, Negri L, Scroppo FI, Grugnetti C (1994) Perineal floor rehabilitation: a new treatment for venogenic impotence. Journal of Endocrinology Investigations 17: 34.

Colpi GM, Negri L, Nappi RE, Chinea B (1999) Perineal floor efficiency in sexually potent and impotent men. International Journal of Impotence Research 11(3): 153–157.

Colpo LM (1998) Evaluation, treatment and management of erectile dysfunction: an overview. Urologic Nursing 18(2): 100–106.

Condra M, Surridge DH, Morales A *et al* (1986) Prevalence and significance of tobacco smoking in impotence. Urology 27: 495–498.

Consensus Statement (1997) First International Conference for the Prevention of Incontinence, 25–27 June 1997, Danesfield House, UK. London: The Continence Foundation.

Davidson PJT, van den Ouden D, Schroeder FH (1996) Radical prostatectomy: prospective assessment of mortality and morbidity. European Urology 29: 168–173.

De Castro R, Ricci G, Gentili A *et al* (1999) Latex allergy in patients who had undergone multiple surgical procedures for urinary bladder exstrophy: preliminary data (abstract). British Journal of Urology International 83 (Suppl 3): 96.

de la Rosette JJMCH, Witjes WPJ, Schäfer W *et al* (1998) Relationships between lower urinary tract symptoms and bladder outlet obstruction: results from the ICS-BPH Study. Neurourology and Urodynamics 17: 99–108.

DeLancey J (1994) Functional anatomy of the pelvic floor and urinary continence mechanism. In: Schüssler B, Laycock J, Norton P, Stanton S (eds) Pelvic Floor Re-education, Principles and Practice. London: Springer-Verlag, pp. 9–21.

Denmeade SR, Lin XS, Isaacs JT (1996) Role of programmed (apoptotic) cell death during the progression and therapy for prostate cancer. Prostate 28: 251–265.

Denning J (1996) Male urinary continence. In: Norton C (ed) Nursing for Continence. Beaconsfield: Beaconsfield, pp. 153–169.

Department of Health (2000) Good Practice in Continence Services. Available from PO Box 777, London SE1 6XH or www.doh.gov.uk/continenceservices.htm

Derouet H, Nolden W, Jost WH *et al* (1998) Treatment of erectile dysfunction by an external ischiocavernosus muscle stimulator. European Urology 34(4): 355–359.

Desai KM, Gingell JC (1989) Hazards of long distance cycling. British Medical Journal 298(6680): 1072–1073.

Dinubile NA (1991) Strength training. Clinical Sports Medicine 10(1): 33–62.

Dixon JS, Gosling JA (1994) The anatomy of the bladder, urethra and pelvic floor. In: Mundy AR, Stephenson TP, Wein AJ (eds) Urodynamics: Principles, Practice and Application (2nd edn). Edinburgh: Churchill Livingstone, pp. 3–14.

Dixon J, Dorey G, Eve B, Simonds K, Taylor V (1997) Post-prostatectomy incontinence. Journal of the Association of Chartered Physiotherapist in Women's Health 80: 35–38.

Djavan B, Madersbacher S, Klinger HC *et al* (1999) Outcome analysis of minimally invasive treatments for benign prostatic hyperplasia. Techniques in Urology 5(1): 12–20.

Djurhuus JC, Matthiesen TB, Rittig S (1999) Similarities and dissimilarities between nocturnal enuresis in childhood and nocturia in adults. British Journal of Urology International 84(Suppl 1): 9–12.

Donnellan SM, Duncan HJ, MacGregor RJ, Russell JM (1997) Prospective assessment of incontinence after radical retropubic prostatectomy: objective and subjective analysis. Urology 49(2): 225–230.

Donovan JL (1999) Measuring the impact of nocturia on quality of life. British Journal of Urology International 84(Suppl 1): 21–25.

Donovan JL, Abrams P, Peters TJ (1996) The ICS-BPH Study: The psychometric validity and reliability of the ICS*male* questionnaire. British Journal of Urology 77: 554–562.

Donovan JL, Kay HE, Peters TJ *et al* (1997) Using ICSQol to measure the impact of lower urinary tract symptoms on quality of life: evidence from the ICS-BPH study. British Journal of Urology 80: 712–721.

Dorey G (1998) Physiotherapy for Male Continence Problems. Physiotherapy 85(11): 556–563.

Dorey G (1999) Physiotherapy for the relief of male lower urinary tract symptoms. Unpublished MSc thesis. University of East London.

Dorey G (2000a) Male patients with lower urinary tract symptoms 1: Assessment. British Journal of Nursing 9(8): 497–501.

Dorey G (2000b) Male patients with lower urinary tract symptoms 2: Treatment. British Journal of Nursing 9(9): 553–558.

Dorey G (2000c) Conservative treatment of erectile dysfunction 1: anatomy/physiology. British Journal of Nursing 9(11): 691–694.

Dorey G (2000d) Conservative treatment of erectile dysfunction 2: clinical trials. British Journal of Nursing 9(12): 755–762.

Dorey G (2000e) Conservative treatment of erectile dysfunction 3: literature review. British Journal of Nursing 9(13): 859–863.

Dorey G (2000f) Physiotherapy for the relief of male lower urinary tract symptoms: A Delphi study. Physiotherapy 86(8): 413–426.

Dorey G (2001a) Is smoking a cause of erectile dysfunction? A review of the literature. British Journal of Nursing 10(7): 455–465.

Dorey G (2001b) Partners' perspective of erectile dysfunction: literature review. British Journal of Nursing 10(3): 187–195.

Drutz HP, Appell RA, Gleason D, Klimberg I, Radomski S (1999) Clinical efficacy and safety of tolterodine compared to oxybutinin and placebo with overactive bladder. International Urogynecology Journal 10: 283–289.

Edmonds SF (1991) Preparing for the return home; discharge information following prostatectomy. Professional Nurse (October): 29–30.

Elbadawi A (1995) Pathology and pathophysiology of the detrusor in incontinence. Urologic Clinics of North America 22: 499–512.

Elbadawi A, Schenk EA (1974) A new theory of the innervation of bladder musculature. Part 4. Innervation of the vesicourethral junction and external urethral sphincter. Journal of Urology 111: 613.

Elder DD, Stephenson TP (1980) An assessment of the Frewen Regime in the treatment of detrusor dysfunction in females. British Journal of Urology 52: 467–471.

Emberton M, Neal DE, Black N et al (1996) The effect of prostatectomy on symptom severity and quality of life. British Journal of Urology 77(2): 233–247.

Emberton M, Meredith P, Wood C et al (1997) An interactive CD-ROM multi-media patient information package for men with lower urinary symptoms. Royal College of Surgeons of England, London UK.

Epstein RS, Deverka PA, Chute CG et al (1992) Validation of a new quality of life questionnaire for benign prostatic hyperplasia. Journal of Clinical Epidemiology 45: 1431–1445.

Fabra M, Porst H (1999) Bulbocavernosus-reflex latencies and pudendal nerve SSEP compared to penile vascular testing in 669 patients with erectile failure and other sexual dysfunction. International Journal of Impotence Research 11(3): 167–175.

Fall M, Lindstrom S (1991) Electrical stimulation: a physiological approach to the treatment of urinary incontinence. Urologic Clinics of North America 18(2): 393–407.

Feldman HA, Goldstein I, Hatzichristou DG et al (1994) Impotence and its medical and psychological correlates: results of the Massachusetts Male Ageing Study. Journal of Urology 151: 54–61.

Fellers CR, Redmon BC, Parrott RN (1933) Effect of cranberries on urinary acidity and blood alkali reserve. Journal of Nutrition 6: 455.

Feneley RCL (1986) Post micturition dribbling. In: Mandelstam D (ed) Incontinence and its Management. London: Croom Helm.

Fisher C, Gross J, Zuch J (1965) Cycle of penile erections synchronous with dreaming (REM) sleep. Archives of General Psychiatry 12: 29–45.

Fletcher EC, Martin RJ (1982) Sexual dysfunction and erectile impotence in chronic obstructive pulmonary disease. Chest 81(4): 413–421.

Fonda D (1999) Nocturia: a disease or normal ageing? British Journal of Urology International 84(Suppl 1): 13–15.

Foote J, Yun S, Leach GE (1991) Post prostatectomy incontinence pathophysiology, evaluation and management. Urologic Clinics of North America 18(2): 229–241.

Fowler FJ Jr, Wennberg JE, Timothy RP et al (1988) Symptom status and quality of life following prostatectomy. Journal of the American Medical Association 259: 3018–3022.

Frewen W (1979) Role of bladder training in the treatment of the unstable bladder in the female. Urologic Clinics of North America 6: 273.

Gambert SR (1997) Alcohol abuse: medical effects of heavy drinking in late life. Geriatrics 52(6): 30–37.

Garraway WM, Collins GN, Lee RJ (1991) High prevalence of benign prostatic hypertrophy in the community. Lancet 338: 469–471.

Garry RC, Roberts TDM, Todd JK (1959) Reflexes involving the external urethral sphincter in the cat. Journal of Physiology 149: 635–65.

Gee WF, Ansell JS, Bonica JJ (1990) Pelvic and perineal pain of urologic origin. In: Bonica JJ (ed) The Management of Pain Vol. 2. Philadelphia: Lea and Febiger, pp. 1368–1394.

Geirsson G, Fall M (1997) Maximal functional electrical stimulation in routine practice. Neurourology and Urodynamics 16: 559–565.

Girman CJ, Epstein RS, Jacobsen SJ et al (1994) Natural history of prostatism: Impact of urinary symptoms on quality of life in 2115 randomly selected community men. Urology 44: 825–831.

Goodson JD (1981) Pudendal neuritis from biking (letter). New England Journal of Medicine 304: 365.

Gordon H, Logue M (1985) Perineal muscle function after childbirth. Lancet 1–2(8441): 123–125.

Gosling JA, Dixon JS, Critchley HOD, Thompson SA (1981) A comparative study of the human external sphincter and periurethral levator ani muscle. British Journal of Urology 53: 35–41.

Gray M (1992) Genitourinary Disorders. Mosby's Clinical Nursing Series. St. Louis, Mo: Mosby, pp. 1–234.

Gray ML (1996) Genitourinary embryology, anatomy and physiology. In: Karlowicz K (ed) Urologic Nursing: Principles and Practice. Philadelphia, Pa: WB Saunders.

Gray ML (1998) Neurophysiology of the bladder. 4th National Multi-speciality Nursing Conference, Orlando, Florida.

Gray ML, Doughty MC (1987) Urinary incontinence: pathophysiology and treatment. Journal of Enterostomal Therapy 14: 152–162.

Griffiths D, Holstege G, Dalm E, Wall H De (1990) Control and coordination of bladder and urethral function in the brain stem of the cat. Neurourology and Urodynamics 9: 63.

Guyton AC (1986) Textbook of Medical Physiology. Philadelphia, Pa: WB Saunders, pp. 1013–1014.

Halaska M, Dorschner W, Frank M (1994) Treatment of urgency and incontinence in elderly patients with propiverine hydrochloride. Neurourology and Urodynamics 13: 428–430.

Hald T, Nordling J, Andersen JT et al (1991) A patient weighted symptom score system in the evaluation of uncomplicated benign prostatic hyperplasia. Scandinavian Journal of Urology and Nephrology (Suppl.) 138: 59–62.

Halloran J (1991) The shared-care model. Medical Journal of Australia 155: 614.

Hansen B, Flyger H, Brasso K et al (1995) Validation of the self-adminstered Danish Prostatic Symptom Score (DAN-PSS-1) system for use in benign prostatic hyperplasia. British Journal of Urology 76: 451–458.

Harrison SCW, Abrams P (1994) Bladder function. In: Sant GR (ed) Pathophysiologic Principles of Urology. Boston, Ma: Blackwell Scientific Publications.

Haslam J (1996) Working together. Nursing Times 92(15): 68.

Haslam EJ (1999) Evaluation of pelvic floor muscle assessment, digital, manometric and surface electromyography in females. Unpublished MPhil Thesis. University of Manchester.

Haslam J, Jeyaseelan S, Oldham JA, Roe BH (1998) Inter-tester reliability for digital assessment of the pelvic floor. 5th Annual Meeting, International Continence Society, UK Section, Cambridge, 2–3 April 1998.

Hayden LJ (1993) Chronic testicular pain. Australian Family Physician 22: 1357–1365.

Helgason AR (1997) Prostate cancer treatment and quality of life – a three level epidemiological approach. Dissertation. Kongliska Carolinska Medico Chirurgiska Institute, Stockholm.

Hirakawa S, Hassouna M, Deleon R, Elhilali M (1993) The role of combined pelvic floor stimulation and biofeedback in post-prostatectomy urinary incontinence (abstract). Journal of Urology 149: 235A.

Holland JM, Feldman JL, Gilbert HC (1994) Phantom orchialgia. Journal of Urology 152: 2291–2293.

Holley RL, Varner RE, Kerns DJ, Mestecky PJ (1995) Long-term failure of pelvic floor musculature exercises in the treatment of genuine stress incontinence. South Medical Journal 88(5): 547–549.

Hunter DJ, Berra-Unamuno A, Martin-Gordo A (1996) Prevalence of urinary symptoms and other urological conditions in Spanish men 50 years old or older. Journal of Urology 155(6): 1965–1970.

ICCC (1998) Interprofessional Collaboration in Continence Care. Nurses and physiotherapists working in continence care. Report of a Consensus Meeting held at the King's Fund, London. London: Association for Continence Advice.

Intili H, Nier D (1998) Self-esteem and depression in men who present with erectile dysfunction. Urologic Nursing 18(3): 185–187.

Jackson J, Emerson L, Johnston B, Wilson J, Morales A (1996) Biofeedback: A noninvasive treatment for incontinence after radical prostatectomy. Urologic Nursing 16(2): 50–54.

Jeremy JY, Mikhailidis DP (1998) Cigarette smoking and erectile dysfunction. Journal of Research in Social Health 118(3): 151–155.

Jolleys JV, Jolleys JCW, Wilson JV *et al* (1993) Does sex equality extend to urinary symptoms? Neurourology and Urodynamics 12: 391–392.

Jones R (1994) Neuromuscular adaptability: therapeutic implications. Journal of the Association of Physiotherapists in Obstetrics and Gynaecology 75: 12–17.

Jones R (1995) Nerves, muscles and continence. Association of Chartered Physiotherapists in Women's Health Annual Conference, 1995, Eastleigh.

Kaplan SA, Santarosa RP, D'Alisera PM *et al* (1997) Pseudodyssynergia (contraction of the external sphincter during voiding) misdiagnosed as chronic nonbacterial prostatitis and the role of biofeedback as a therapeutic option. Journal of Urology 157: 2234–2237.

Karpukhin IV, Bogomol'nyi VA (1999) Physical factors in the treatment and rehabilitation of patients with chronic prostatitis complicated by impotence (in Russian). Voprosy Kurortologii Fizioterapii I Lechebnoi Fizicheskoi Kultury (Moskva) 2: 25–27.

Kawanishi Y, Yamaguchi K, Kishimoto T *et al* (2000) Simple evaluation of ischiocavernosus muscle. International Journal of Impotence Research 12(Suppl 2): S13.

Kegel AH (1956) Early genital relaxation. Obstetrics and Gynecology 8(5): 545–550.

Kho HG, Sweep CG, Chen X, Rabsztyn PR, Meuleman EJ (1999) The use of acupuncture in the treatment of erectile dysfunction. International Journal of Impotence Research 11(1): 41–46.

Kinney AB, Blount M (1979) Effect of cranberry juice on urinary pH. Nursing Research 28(5): 287–290.

Kirby R, Fitzpatrick J, Kirby M, Fitzpatrick A (ed.) (1994) Shared Care for Prostatic Diseases. Oxford: Isis Medical Media, p. 16.

Kirby R, Carson C, Goldstein I (1999) Anatomy, physiology and pathophysiology. In: Kirby R (ed) Erectile Dysfunction: A Clinical Guide. Oxford: Isis Medical Media, pp. 11–28.

Knight SJ, Laycock J (1994) The role of biofeedback in pelvic floor re-education. Physiotherapy 80: 145–148.

Knight SJ, Laycock J (1998) Evaluation of neuromuscular electrical stimulation in the treatment of genuine stress incontinence. Physiotherapy 84(2): 61–71.

Koeman M, Van Driel MF, Weijmar Schultz WCM, Mensink HJA (1996) Orgasm after radical prostatectomy. British Journal of Urology 77: 861–864.

Kortmann BBM, Sonke GS, D'Ancona FCH *et al* (1999) The tolerability of urodynamic studies and flexible cystourethroscopy used in the assessment of men with lower urinary tract symptoms. British Journal of Urology 84: 449–453.

Kosch SG, Curry RW Jr, Kuritzky L (1988) Evaluation and treatment of impotence: a pragmatic approach addressing organic and psychogenic components. Family Practitioner Research Journal 7(3): 162–174.

Krane RJ, Goldstein I, Sáenz Tejada I De (1989) Medical progress: impotence. New England Journal of Medicine 321: 1648–1659.

Krauss DJ, Lilien OM (1981) Transcutaneous electrical nerve stimulator for stress incontinence. Journal of Urology 125: 790–793.

La Pera G, Nicastro A (1996) A new treatment for premature ejaculation: the rehabilitation of the pelvic floor. Journal of Sex and Marital Therapy 22(1): 22–26.

Lavoisier P, Courtois F, Barres D, Blanchard M (1986) Correlation between intracavernous pressure and contraction of the ischiocavernosus muscle in man. Journal of Urology 136: 936–939.

Lavoisier P, Proulz J, Courtois F, Carufel F De, Durand L (1988) Relationship between perineal muscle contractions, penile tumescence, and penile rigidity during nocturnal erections. Journal of Urology 139: 176–179.

Lavoisier P, Schmidt M, Alaoui R (1992) Intracavernous pressure increases and perineal muscle contractions in response to pressure stimulation of the glans penis. International Journal of Impotence Research 4: 157.

Lawrence WT, MacDonagh RP (1988) Treatment of urethral stricture disease by internal urethrotomy followed by intermittent 'low friction' self-catheterisation. Journal of the Royal Society of Medicine 81(3): 136–139.

Laycock J (1994) Female pelvic floor assessment: the Laycock ring of continence. Journal of the National Women 's Health Group, Australian Physiotherapy Association 13: 40–51.

Laycock J, Plevnick S, Senn E (1994) Electrical stimulation. In: Schüssler B, Laycock J, Norton P, Stanton S (eds) Pelvic Floor Re-education: Principles and practice. London: Springer-Verlag, pp. 143–153.

Le Lievre S (1999) Care of the incontinent client's skin. Journal of Community Nursing 14(2): 26–32.

Leaver RB (1996) Cranberry juice. Professional Nurse 11(8): 525–526.

Lepor H, Grace M (1993) Comparison of AUA symptom index in unselected males and females between 55 and 79 years of age. Urology 42: 36–40.

Levin RM, Wein AJ (1995) Neurophysiology and neuropharmacology. In: Fitzpatrick JM, Krane RJ (eds) The Bladder. London: Churchill Livingstone, pp. 47–70.

Lewis RW, Mills TM (1999) Risk factors for impotence. In: Carson CC, Kirby RS, Goldstein I (eds) Textbook of Erectile Dysfunction. Oxford: Isis Medical Media, pp. 141–8.

Light JK, Rapoll E, Wheeler TM (1997) The striated urethral sphincter: muscle fibre types and distribution in the prostatic capsule. British Journal of Urology 79: 539–542.

Lizza EF, Rosen RC (1999) Definition and classification of erectile dysfunction: Report of the Nomenclature Committee of the International Society of Impotence Research. International Journal of Impotence Research 11(3): 141–143.

Lombardi G (1999) Reprogrammation sensitivo mortice dans le syndrome de l'éjaculation prematée. Conference proceedings, Premières recontres méditérranéennes d'actualités thérapeutiques réhabilitatives sur les dysfonctions du plancher pelvien, 19–21 Novembre 1999, Marseille.

LoPiccolo J (1986) Diagnosis and treatment of male sexual dysfunction. Journal of Marital Therapy 11: 215–232.

Madsen PO, Iversen P (1983) A point system for selecting operative candidates. In: Hinman F (ed) Benign Prostatic Hypertrophy. New York: Springer-Verlag, pp. 763–765.

Mahady IW, Begg BM (1981) Long term symptomatic and cystometric care of the urge incontinence syndrome using a technique of bladder re-education. British Journal of Obstetrics and Gynecology 88: 1038–1043.

Mahony DT, Laferte RO, Blais DJ (1977) Integral storage and voiding reflexes. Neurology 9(1): 95–106.

Malmsten UGH, Milsom I, Molander U, Norlen LJ (1997) Urinary incontinence and lower urinary tract symptoms: an epidemiological study of men aged 45 to 99 years. Journal of Urology 158: 1733–1737.

Malone-Lee JG (2000) The efficacy, tolerability and safety profile of tolterodine in the treatment of overactive/unstable bladder. Reviews in Contemporary Pharmacotherapy 11: 29–42.

Mamberti-Dias A, Bonierbale-Branchereau M (1991) Therapy for dysfunctioning erections: four years later, how do things stand?. Sexologique 1: 24–25.

Mamberti-Dias A, Vasavada SP, Bourcier AP (1999) Pelvic floor dysfunction; investigations and conservative treatment. Paris: Casa Editrice Scientifica Internationale, pp. 303–310.

Mannino DM, Klevens RM, Flanders WD (1994) Cigarette smoking: an independent risk factor for impotence? American Journal of Epidemiology 140(11): 1003–1008.

Mathewson-Chapman M (1997) Pelvic muscle exercise/biofeedback for urinary incontinence after prostatectomy: an education program. Journal of Cancer Education 12(4): 218–223.

McArdle WD, Catch FI, Catch VL (1991) Exercise Physiology (2nd edn). Philadelphia: Lea and Febinger, pp. 1–12.

McGuire EJ, O'Connell HE (1995) The bladder and spinal cord injury. In: Fitzpatrick JM, Krane RJ (ed) The Bladder. New York: Churchill Livingstone, pp. 213–227.

Meaglia JP, Joseph AC, Chang M, Schmidt JD (1990) Post-prostatectomy urinary incontinence: response to behavioral training. Journal of Urology 144(3): 674–676.

Meehan JP, Goldstein AMB (1983) High pressure within corpus cavernosum in man during erection. Its probable mechanism. Urology 21: 385.

Mellion MB (1991) Common cycling injuries. Management and prevention. Sports Medicine 11(1): 52–72.

Melman A, Gingell JC (1999) The epidemiology and pathophysiology of erectile dysfunction. Journal of Urology 161(1): 5–11.

Michal V, Simana J, Rehak J, Masim J (1983) Haemodynamics of erection in man. Physiologia Bohemoslovaca 32: 497.

Middlekoop HAM, Smilde-van den Doel DA, Neven AK, Kamphuisen HAC, Springer CP (1996) Subjective sleep characteristics of 1,485 males and females aged 50–93; Effect of sex and age and factors related to self-evaluated quality of sleep. Journal of Gerontology 51A: 108–115.

Mikhailidis DP, Ganotakis ES, Papadakis JA, Jeremy JY (1998) Smoking and urological disease. Journal of the Royal Society of Health 118(4): 210–212.

Millard RJ (1989) After-dribble. Bladder Control – A simple Self-help Guide. NSW, Australia: William & Wilkins, pp. 89–90.

Millard RJ, Oldenburg BF (1983) The symptomatic, urodynamic and psychodynamic results of bladder re-education programs. Journal of Urology 130: 715–719.

Milne JS, Williamson J, Maule MM (1972) Urinary symptoms in older people. Modern Geriatrics 2: 198–212.

Moen DV (1962) Observations on the effectiveness of cranberry juice in urinary infections. Wisconsin Medical Journal 61: 282–283.

Moncada Iribarren I, Sáenz Tejada I de (1999) Vascular physiology of penile erection. In: Carson CC, Kirby RS, Goldstein I (eds) Textbook of Erectile Dysfunction. Oxford: Isis Medical Media.

Moore H (1990) Caffeine. Which? (June): 314–317.

Moore KN (1997) Conservative management of urinary incontinence post radical prostatectomy: impact of urine loss and health-related quality of life. Unpublished Doctoral thesis, Faculty of Nursing. University of Alberta, Edmonton, Canada.

Moore KN, Dorey G (1999) Conservative treatment of urinary incontinence in men: A review of the literature. Physiotherapy 85(2): 77–87.

Moore KN, Griffiths DJ, Hughton A (1999) A randomised controlled trial comparing pelvic muscle exercises with pelvic muscle exercises plus electrical stimulation for the treatment of post-prostatectomy urinary incontinence. British Journal of Urology 83: 57–65.

Moul JW (1994) For incontinence after prostatectomy, tap a diversity of treatments. Contemporary Urology (April): 78–88.

Moul JW (1998) Pelvic muscle rehabilitation in males following prostatectomy. Urologic Nursing 18(4): 296–301.

Narayan P, Konety B, Aslam K *et al* (1995) Neuroanatomy of the external urethral sphincter: implications for urinary continence preservation during radical prostatectomy surgery. Journal of Urology 153: 337–341.

Nayal W, Schwarzer U, Klotz T, Heidenreich A, Engelmann U (1999) Transcutaneous penile oxygen pressure during bicycling. British Journal of Urology International 83(6): 623–625.

Neal DE (1990) Prostatectomy – an open and closed case. British Journal of Urology 66: 449–454.

Neal DE (1997) The National Prostatectomy Audit. British Journal of Urology 79(2): 69–75.

Nickel JC for the Canadian PROSPECT Group (1998) PROscar Safety Efficiency Canadian Two year study on Proscar (prspect) group. Placebo therapy of benign prostatic hyperplasia: a 25-month study. British Journal of Urology 81: 383–387.

NIH (1993) National Institutes of Health Consensus Development Panel on Impotence. Journal of the American Medical Association 270: 83–90.

Norris C (1997) Muscle training/muscle imbalance. 4th Biennial Pelvic Floor Conference, 1–2 December 1997, Harrogate.

O'Farrell TJ, Kleinke CL, Cutter HS (1998) Sexual adjustment of male alcoholics: changes from before to after receiving alcoholism counselling with and without marital therapy. Addictive Behaviour 23(3): 419–425.

O'Leary MP, Fowler FJ, Lenderking WR *et al* (1995) A brief male sexual function inventory for urology. Urology 46: 697–706.

Office of Health Economics (1995) Diseases of the Prostate. Luton: White Crescent Press.

OPCS (1996) Population Trends. No. 85, Autumn. London: Office of Population Censuses and Surveys.

Palermo LM, Zimskind PD (1977) Effect of caffeine on urethral presure. Urology 10(4): 320–324.

Park JM, Bloom DA, McGuire EJ (1997) The guarding reflex revisited. British Journal of Urology 80: 940–945.

Paterson J, Pinnock CB, Marshall VR (1997) Pelvic floor exercises as a treatment for post-micturition dribble. British Journal of Urology 79: 892–897.

Paulson DF (1991) Editorial comments. Journal of Urology 145: 515.

Pettersson L, Fader M (2000) An evaluation of all-in-one incontinence pads. Nursing Times Plus 96(6): 11.

Pinnock CB, Stapleton AM, Marshall VR (1999) Erectile dysfunction in the community: a prevalence study. Medical Journal of Australia 171(7): 353–357.

Poirier P, Charpy A (1901) Traite d'anatomie humaine. Paris: Masson, pp. 197–201.

Pomfret I (1993) Male incontinence. Community Outlook (March): 45.

Pomfret I (1996) The use of continence products. In: Norton C (ed) Nursing for Continence (2nd edn). Beaconsfield: Beaconsfield Publishers, pp. 335–364.

Porru D, Campus G, Caria A *et al* (2001) Impact of early pelvic floor rehabilitation after transurethral resection of prostate. Neurourology and Urodynamics 20: 53–59.

Ramsden P, Hindmarsh J, Bowditch J *et al* (1982) DDAVP for adult enuresis – a preliminary report. British Journal of Urology 54: 256.

Resnick MI (1992) Carcinoma of the prostate. In: Resnick MI, Caldamone AA Spirnak JP, Decker BC (ed) Decision Making in Urology. Philadelphia: BC Decker, pp. 114–115.

Robert R, Brunet C, Faure A *et al* (1993) La chirurgie du nerf pudental lors de certaines algies perineales: evolution et resultats. Chirurgie 119: 535–539.

Rogers J (1991) Pass the cranberry juice. Nursing Times 87(48): 36–37.

Rosen RC, Riley A, Wagner G et al (1997) The international index of erectile function (IIEF): a multidimensional scale for assessment of erectile dysfunction. Urology 49(6): 822–830.

Royal Commission on the NHS (1978) Patients' Attitudes to Hospital Services. London: Royal Commission on the NHS.

Rudy DC, Woodside JR, Crawford ED (1984) Urodynamic evaluation of incontinence in patients undergoing modified Campbell radical retro pubic prostatectomy: A prospective study. Journal of Urology 132: 708–712.

Salmons S, Henriksonn J (1981) The adaptive response of skeletal muscle to increased use. Muscle and Nerve 4: 94–105.

Sant GR, Long JP (1994) Benign prostatic hyperplasia. In: Sant GR (ed) Pathophysiologic Principles of Urology. Blackwell Scientific Publications, London, pp. 123–154.

Scafer W, Nopponey R, Rabben H, Lutzeyer W (1988) The value of free flow rate and pressure flow studies in the routine investigation of BPH patients. Neurourology and Urodynamics 7: 219–221.

Schouman M, Lacroix P (1991) Apport de la ré-éducation pelvi-périnéale au traitement des fuites veino-caverneuses. Annales Urologique 25: 92–93.

Segura JW, Opitz JL, Greene LF (1979) Prostatosis, prostatitis or pelvic floor tension myalgia? Journal of Urology 122: 168–169.

Shabsigh R, Fishman IJ, Schum C, Dunn JK (1991) Cigarette smoking and other vascular risk factors in vasculogenic impotence. Urology 38(3): 227–231.

Shafik A (1996) Extrapelvic cavernous nerve stimulation in erectile dysfunction. Human study. Andrologia 28(3): 151–156.

Simpson RJ, Fisher W, Lee AJ, Russell EBAW, Garraway M (1996) Benign prostatic hyperplasia in an unselected community-based population: a survey of urinary symptoms, bothersomeness and prostatic enlargement. British Journal of Urology 77: 186–191.

Singh NP, Sharp A, Ferro MA (1997) Pulsed short-wave therapy for chronic prostatitis (abstract). British Journal of Urology 79 (Suppl 4): 69.

Siroky MB (1996) Electromyography of the perineal floor. Urologic Clinics of North America 23(2): 299–307.

Smith M (1997) Trickle of information. Nursing Times Supplement 93: 5.

Solomon S, Cappa KG (1987) Impotence and bicycling. A seldom-reported connection. Postgraduate Medicine 81(1): 99–100.

Sotiropoulos A, Yeaw S, Lattimer JK (1976) Management of urinary incontinence with electronic stimulation: Observations and results. Journal of Urology 116: 747–750.

Steers WD (1992) Physiology of the urinary bladder. In: Walsh PC, Retik AB, Stamey TA, Vaughan ED Jr (eds) Campbell's Urology. Philadelphia: WB Saunders, pp. 142–178.

Stief CG, Weller E, Noack T et al (1996) Functional electromyostimulation of the penile corpus cavernosum (FEMCC). Initial results of a new therapeutic option of erectile dysfunction. Urologe A 35(4): 321–325.

Strasser H, Steinlechner M, Bartsch G (1997) Morphometric analysis of the rhabdosphincter of the male urethra. Journal of Urology 157(Suppl 4): 177.

Sueppel C (1998) Timing of pelvic floor muscle strengthening exercises and return of continence in post prostatectomy patients. 4th National Multi-Specialty Nursing Conference on Urinary Continence, 1998, Florida. Society of Urologic Nurses and Associates.

Tan RS, Philip PS (1999) Perceptions of and risk factors for andropause. Archives of Andrology 43(3): 227–233.

Tanagho EA (1990) Electrical Stimulation. Journal of the American Geriatrics Society 38: 352–355.

Thomas TM, Plymat KR, Blannin J, Meade TW (1980) The prevalence of urinary incontinence. British Medical Journal 281: 1243–1245.

Torrens M (1987) Human physiology. In: Torrens M, Morrison JFB (eds) Physiology of the Lower Urinary Tract. London: Springer-Verlag, pp. 33–350.

Trueman P, Hood SC, Nayak USL, Mrazek MF (1999) Prevalence of lower urinary tract symptoms and self-reported diagnosed 'benign prostatic hyperplasia', and their effect on quality of life in a community-based survey of men in the UK. British Journal of Urology International 83: 410–415.

Van Kampen M (1998) Male incontinence and impotence. Unpublished PhD thesis. Katholieke Universiteit Leuven, Belgium.

Van Kampen M, Weerdt W De, Poppel H Van et al (2000) Effect of pelvic floor re-education on duration and degree of incontinence after radical prostatectomy: a randomised controlled trial. Lancet 355(9198): 98–102.

Van Kerrebroeck P, Weiss J (1999) Standardization and terminology of nocturia. British Journal of Urology International 84(Suppl 1): 1–4.

Vereecken RL, Wouters M (1988) Discrepancies between clinical and urodynamic findings: Which are true? Urology International 43: 282.

Vestey SB, Hinchcliffe A (1998) The frequency/volume (F/V) chart: don't be without one! British Journal of Urology 81(Suppl 4): 21.

Vidal Moreno JF, Moreno Pardo B, Jimenez Cruz JF (1996) Assessment of tobacco impact on penile vascularization with echo-Doppler and intracavernous injection. Actas Urologicas Espanolas 20(4): 365–371.

Wagg A, Malone-Lee J (1999) Problems in elderly people. In: Wagg A, Malone-Lee J (ed) Bladder Problems. London: Martin Dunitz, pp. 44–51.

Wagner TH, Patrick DL, McKenna SP Froese PS (1996) Cross-cultural development of a quality of life measure for men with erection difficulties. Quality of Life Research 5: 443–449.

Wein AW (1997) Pharmacologic options for the overactive bladder. Urology 51(Suppl 2A): 43–47.

Weisberg HF (1982) Water, Electrolyte and Acid-base Balance (2nd edn). Baltimore, Md.: Williams & Wilkins.

Weiss JP, Stember DS, Blaivas JG, Brooks MM (1998) Nocturia in adults: classification and etiology. Neurourology and Urodynamics 17: 467–472.

Wells TJ (1988) Additional treatments for urinary incontinence. Topics in Geriatric Rehabilitation 3(2): 48–57.

Wespes E, Nogueira MC, Herbaut AG, Caufriez M, Schulman CC (1990) Role of the bulbocavernosus muscles on the mechanism of human erection. European Urology 18: 45–48.

Wesselmann U, Burnett AL, Heinberg LJ (1997) The urogenital and rectal pain syndromes. Pain 73: 269–294.

Wetterling T, Veltrup C, Driessen M, John U (1999) Drinking pattern and alcohol-related medical disorders. Alcohol and Alcoholism 34(3): 330–336.

Wheelahan J, Scott NA, Cartmill R et al (The ASERNIP-S review group) (2000) Minimally invasive non-laser thermal techniques for prostatectomy: a systematic review. British Journal of Urology International 86: 977–988.

Wilson DP, Al Samarrai T, Deakin M, Kolbe E, Brown ADG (1987) An objective assessment of physiotherapy for female genuine stress incontinence. British Journal of Obstetrics and Gynaecology 94: 575–582.

World Health Organization (1978) Definition of Health. Geneva, Switzerland: WHO.

Index